Nutrition and Health

Nutrition and Health

Web Resource Guide for Consumers,
Healthcare Providers, Patients and
Physicians

Eugene A. DeFelice, M.D.

iUniverse, Inc.
New York Lincoln Shanghai

Nutrition and Health
Web Resource Guide for Consumers, Healthcare Providers, Patients and Physicians

iUniverse, Inc.

For information address:
iUniverse, Inc.
2021 Pine Lake Road, Suite 100
Lincoln, NE 68512
www.iuniverse.com

ISBN: 0-595-29675-0 (pbk)
ISBN: 0-595-75114-8 (cloth)

Printed in the United States of America

This book is dedicated to Ms. Maryanne Harvey, M.S. and Mr. Benjamin DeFelice.

Maryanne, my friend, has devoted most of her professional life to the betterment of the health and welfare of others as a member of the New York State Department of Health, which she now serves as a consultant. Without Maryanne's able professional advice and assistance, publication of this book would not have been possible.

Ben, my brother, world traveler, raconteur extraordinaire, friend and helping hand to many throughout his life, a "man for all seasons", served as my Literary Agent regarding publication of this book.

Contents

Preface. xvii

1. Basic Nutrition Guidelines 1

- *1.1 Introduction* *1*
- *1.2 Dietary Reference Intakes (DRIs)* *3*
- *1.3 Essential Vitamins/Minerals DRIs* *6*
- *1.4 Energy Nutrients* *8*
- *1.5 Carbohydrates* *10*
- *1.6 Proteins* *10*
- *1.7 Fats* *12*
- *1.8 Trans Fats* *13*
- *1.8.1. Introduction* *13*
- *1.8.2 Reducing Dietary Trans Fats* *14*
- *1.8.3 Trans Fat Food Labeling* *17*
- *1.9 Dietary Fiber* *18*
- *1.9.1 Introduction* *18*
- *1.9.2 Recommended Fiber Intake* *19*
- *1.9.3 Benefits of Dietary Fiber* *19*
- *1.10 Fish/Fish Oils* *21*
- *1.11 Flaxseed/Flaxseed Oils* *26*

2. Dietary Guidelines for Americans. 28

- *2.1 Introduction* *28*
- *2.2 ABCs of Dietary Guidelines* *28*
- *2.3 Aim for fitness* *29*
- *2.4 Build A Healthy Base/Food Guide Pyramid* *31*

- *2.5 Choose a Sensible Diet* *32*
- *2.6 Mediterranean Diet/Pyramid* *36*
- *2.7 AHA Dietary Guidelines* *37*
- *2.8 Dr. Atkins Diet* *38*
- *2.9 Dr. Ornish Diet* *39*
- *2.10 Moderate Fat Diet* *40*

3. Phytonutrients/Phytochemicals 42
- *3.1 Introduction* *42*
- *3.2 Disease Prevention Mechanisms* *44*
- *3.3 Potential Health Benefits* *45*
- *3.4 Increasing Phytonutrient Intake* *46*
- *3.5 Major Classes of Phytonutrients* *47*
- *3.5.1 Carotenoids* *48*
- *3.5.2 Phenolic acids* *51*
- *3.5.3 Flavonoids/Polyphenols* *52*
- *3.5.4 Sulfur Containing Compounds* *54*
- *3.5.4.1 Indoles* *54*
- *3.5.4.2 Sulforaphane/Glucosinolates* *54*
- *3.5.4.3 Isothiocyanates* *55*
- *3.5.4.4 Thiosulfonates* *55*
- *3.5.4.5 Terpenes* *56*
- *3.5.5 Phytosterols* *56*
- *3.5.6 Phytoestrogens/Isoflavones* *57*
- *3.6 Whole Grain Phytonutrients* *58*
- *3.7 Flaxseed Phytonutrients* *61*
- *3.8 Phytonutrients/Cancer Prevention* *62*

4. Five to Nine a Day: Fruits/Vegetables/Seeds/Nuts 64
- *4.1 Introduction* *64*
- *4.2 Research Backs Benefits* *65*
- *4.3 Color Your Way/5 to 9 a Day* *66*
- *4.3.1 Introduction* *66*
- *4.3.2 Blues/Purples* *66*
- *4.3.3 Greens* *67*
- *4.3.4 Oranges/Yellows* *68*

- *4.3.5 Reds/Pinks* *70*
- *4.3.6 Whites/Browns/Tans* *71*
- *4.4 Fruits/Vegetables* *72*
- *4.4.1 Apples* *73*
- *4.4.2 Asparagus* *74*
- *4.4.3 Bananas* *75*
- *4.4.4 Beets* *75*
- *4.4.5 Berries* *76*
- *4.4.5.1 Introduction* *76*
- *4.4.5.2 Blackberries* *77*
- *4.4.5.3 Blueberries* *77*
- *4.4.5.4 Cranberries* *79*
- *4.4.5.5 Raspberries* *80*
- *4.4.5.6 Strawberries* *82*
- *4.4.6 Broccoli* *84*
- *4.4.7 Brussels Sprouts* *86*
- *4.4.8 Cabbage* *86*
- *4.4.9 Carrots* *87*
- *4.4.10 Cauliflower* *88*
- *4.4.11 Celery* *89*
- *4.4.12 Cherries* *90*
- *4.4.13 Corn* *93*
- *4.4.14 Dried Beans* *94*
- *4.4.15 Figs* *95*
- *4.4.16 Grapefruit* *96*
- *4.4.17 Grapes/Raisins/Grape Juice/Wine* *97*
- *4.4.17.1 Grapes* *97*
- *4.4.17.2 Raisins* *98*
- *4.4.17.3 Grape Juice* *99*
- *4.4.17.4 Wine* *99*
- *4.4.18 Kiwis* *101*
- *4.4.19 Lemons* *102*
- *4.4.20 Lentils/Dried Peas/Chickpeas/Soybeans* *103*
- *4.4.20.1 Lentils* *103*
- *4.4.20.2 Dried Peas* *104*

- *4.4.20.3 Chickpeas* *104*
- *4.4.20.4 Soybeans* *105*
- *4.4.21 Mangos* *109*
- *4.4.22 Mushrooms* *109*
- *4.4.23 Onions* *110*
- *4.4.24 Oranges* *111*
- *4.4.25 Papayas* *112*
- *4.4.26 Passion Fruits* *113*
- *4.4.27 Peaches* *114*
- *4.4.28 Pears* *115*
- *4.4.29 Peas/Fresh* *116*
- *4.4.30 Peppers/Bell* *117*
- *4.4.31 Pineapples* *118*
- *4.4.32 Plums/Prunes* *118*
- *4.4.33 Squash* *121*
- *4.4.34 Sweet Potatoes* *122*
- *4.4.35 Tomatoes* *123*
- *4.4.36 Watermelons* *124*
- *4.5 Seeds/Nuts* *126*
- *4.5.1. Introduction* *126*
- *4.5.2 Walnuts* *127*
- *4.5.3 Peanuts* *129*
- *4.5.4 Chestnuts* *130*

5. Dietary Supplements 131
- *5.1 Introduction* *131*
- *5.2 Classification of Ingredients* *131*
- *5.3 FDA Regulation/Labeling* *132*
- *5.4 Tips/Dietary Supplement Users* *133*
- *5.5 Dietary Supplement Claims* *133*
- *5.6 Advertisement Regulation* *135*
- *5.7 Adverse Events Reporting* *135*
- *5.8 Recent Information on Dietary Supplements* *135*
- *5.9 Center for Food Safety and Applied Nutrition* *135*
- *5.10 Potential Health Benefits* *136*
- *5.10.1 Fish/Flaxseed/Oils* *137*

- *5.10.2 Niacin* *137*
- *5.10.3 Stress Tabs* *137*
- *5.10.4 Antioxidants/Vitamins* *138*
- *5.10.5 Vitamin D* *139*
- *5.10.6 Folate* *140*
- *5.10.7 Vitamin B-12* *140*
- *5.10.8 Garlic* *140*
- *5.10.9 Chromium* *141*
- *5.10.10 Magnesium* *141*
- *5.10.11 Potassium* *141*
- *5.10.12 Calcium* *142*
- *5.10.13 Multivitamin/Mineral* *142*
- *5.10.14 Tea* *142*
- *5.10.15 Plant Sterols/Stanols* *145*

6. Essential Vitamins/Minerals 147
- *6.1 Introduction* *147*
- *6.2 Fat soluble Vitamins* *149*
- *6.2.1 Vitamin A (Retinol/Beta Carotene)* *149*
- *6.2.2 Vitamin D (Calciferol)* *152*
- *6.2.3 Vitamin E (Tocopherols)* *154*
- *6.2.4 Vitamin K (phylloquinone)* *156*
- *6.3 Water soluble Vitamins* *158*
- *6.3.1 Vitamin C (Ascorbic Acid)* *159*
- *6.3.2 Biotin* *162*
- *6.3.3 Choline* *164*
- *6.3 4 Vitamin B-1 (Thiamine)* *167*
- *6.3.5 Vitamin B-2 (Riboflavin)* *169*
- *6.3.6 Vitamin B-3 (Niacin)* *171*
- *6.3.7 Vitamin B-5 (Pantothenic Acid)* *173*
- *6.3.8 Vitamin B-6 (Pyridoxine)* *175*
- *6.3.9 Vitamin B-9 (Folate/Folic Acid)* *176*
- *6.3.10 Vitamin B-12 (Cobalamin)* *177*
- *6.4 Major Minerals* *179*
- *6.4.1 Calcium* *179*
- *6.4.2 Magnesium* *183*

- 6.4.3 Phosphorous 185
- 6.5 Mineral Electrolytes.. 187
- 6.5.1 Sodium/Chloride (Salt)..................................... 187
- 6.5.2 Potassium 190
- 6.6 Trace Minerals... 193
- 6.6.1 Chromium 193
- 6.6.2 Cobalt... 195
- 6.6.3 Copper 196
- 6.6.4 Fluorine 198
- 6.6.5 Iodine 200
- 6.6.6 Iron... 202
- 6.6.7 Manganese 204
- 6.6.8 Molybdenum... 204
- 6.6.9 Selenium.. 205
- 6.6.10 Zinc 207
- 6.7 Unclassified Trace Minerals.................................. 209
- 6.7.1 Boron 209
- 6.8 Multiple Vitamin/Mineral Supplement....................... 210

7. Author's List/Key Web Sources............................... 213
- 7.1 AlltheWeb 213
- 7.2 American Dietetic Association 214
- 7.3 American Heart Association................................... 215
- 7.4 American Medical Association 215
- 7.5 Food and Drug Administration............................... 215
- 7.6 Food Standards Agency 216
- 7.7 Google.com... 216
- 7.8 Harvard School of Public Health 216
- 7.9 Health.gov... 217
- 7.10 Health on the Net Foundation.............................. 218
- 7.11 Institute of Medicine 219
- 7.12 Iowa State University/Extension 219
- 7.13 Mayo Clinic.. 220
- 7.14 Medline 220
- 7.15 Medlineplus.. 221
- 7.16 National Cancer Institute 221

- *7.17 National Center for Chronic Disease Prevention and Health Promotion* *222*
- *7.18 National Institute on Aging* *222*
- *7.19 National Institutes of Health* *223*
- *7.20 National Institute of Health/Clinical Center* *223*
- *7.21 National Library of Medicine*.................................... *224*
- *7.22 Nutrition.Gov.*.. *224*
- *7.23 Nutrition.Org/American Society for Nutritional Sciences* *225*
- *7.24 Office of Dietary Supplements*................................... *225*
- *7.25 Tufts Nutritional Navigator*..................................... *226*
- *7.26 USDA Center for Nutrition Policy Promotion* *227*
- *7.27 USDA Food and Nutrition Information Center*...................... *228*
- *7.28 USDA Nutrient Data Laboratory/Agricultural Research Service*.......... *229*
- *7.29 USDA Phytonutrient Laboratory*................................. *231*
- *7.30 WebMD* *232*

8. Searching the Web 233

About the Author 237

Acknowledgements

The author acknowledges that the Web Resources listed in Chapter 7, Author's List/Key Web Resources, and additional ones cited in the text, provided the information on nutrition and health presented in this book. The author also wishes to thank the J. Spencer and Patricia Standish Library of Siena College, in Loudonville, New York for the use of their library/computer facilities and assistance provided in researching the subject matter for the book.

Preface

Most individuals do not devote sufficient attention to good nutrition and health. Rather they tend to:

> Squander health in search of wealth
> They work and toil and save
> Then squander wealth in search of health
> But find an early grave.
>
> Anonymous

The US Surgeon General's Report on "Nutrition and Health" in 1988 noted that roughly two thirds of all deaths are due to chronic diseases associated with diet, especially cancers and cardiovascular diseases.

Four of the most important personal habits that influence health are smoking, alcohol consumption, lack of exercise, and diet. For two out of three adults who do not drink alcohol in excess or smoke, the two most important choices influencing long term health are nutrition (diet) and exercise, and nutrition appears to be the most important.

In 1997, the World Cancer Research Fund, and the American Institute for Cancer Research report entitled, "Food, Nutrition, and the Prevention of Cancer: A Global Perspective", stated that recommended diets in conjunction with physical activity and normal weight (body mass index) could reduce cancer by up to 40%.

Regarding cardiovascular disease, the 1989 National Academy of Science report "Diet and Health: Implications for Reducing Chronic Disease Risk" projected that a very large number of all deaths could be avoided by reducing fats, and increasing fruits, vegetables, whole grain breads and cereals, and legumes (dry beans, lentils and peas) in the diet.

Unfortunately, most adult Americans apparently have yet to adopt good nutrition and a healthy lifestyle to avoid chronic disease and premature death. Nevertheless, there is still time for all concerned to heed the call.

This book is a useful state-of-the-art review of available information on the subject, and a guide to key Web Resources by which to obtain current, comprehensive, reliable and useful information on nutrition and health. Bear in mind, however, that in order to become properly informed and knowledgeable, and assume responsibility, one needs to ask the right questions and obtain the best information available. In this regard, it has been said:

> I keep six honest serving men
> They taught me all I knew
> Their names are What and Why and When
> And How and Where and Who.
>
> Rudyard Kipling

Chapter 1 provides information on Basic Nutrition Guidelines, Chapter 2 on Dietary Guidelines for Americans, Chapter 3 on Phytonutrients/Phytochemicals, Chapter 4 on 5 to 9 a Day/Fruits/Vegetables/Seeds/Nuts, Chapter 5 on Dietary Supplements, Chapter 6 on Essential Vitamins/Minerals, Chapter 7 on Author's List/Key Web Resources, and Chapter 8 on Searching the Web.

With the information obtained from this book and the Web, one may become informed, take responsibility for their nutrition and health, make informed decisions with their physician/healthcare provider, and live a healthier, happier, longer, and more productive/enjoyable life. In so doing, remember that:

> Nutrition is not what it used to be.
> Nutrition is not even what it ought to be.
> Nutrition on the Web has grown to be.
> Nutrition available to all as it should be.
>
> Eugene A. DeFelice, MD

Individuals should bear in mind that there is no one best answer for any question regarding nutrition and health. Rather, one must ultimately obtain the best information available from a variety of sources, and decide what is "right/best" under the particular circumstances of the moment in conjunction with their physician/health care provider.

Eugene A. DeFelice, MD

1. Basic Nutrition Guidelines

1.1 Introduction

The latest report from the Institute of Medicine (IOM), Food and Nutrition Board (FNB) recommends that adults obtain 45 to 65% of their calories from carbohydrates, 20 to 35% from fat, and 10 to 35% from protein in order to meet the body's daily energy and nutritional needs, while minimizing the risk for chronic disease. When caloric intake is increased, a high fat diet can lead to overweight, obesity, and health related complications such as diabetes mellitus (non-insulin-dependent type 2), and increases in low density lipoprotein cholesterol (LDL-C or "bad" cholesterol) and cardiovascular disease. On the other hand, very low fat and high carbohydrate diets can lead to decreases in high density lipoprotein cholesterol (HDL-C or "good" cholesterol) also increasing susceptibility to cardiovascular disease.

Sound nutrition is essential to good health and longevity. A United States Department of Agriculture (USDA) report provides basic considerations for sound nutrition at:
http://www.ars.usda.gov/is/np/fnrb/fnrb/197.htm

IOM/FNB stresses the importance of balancing total calories consumed with appropriate physical activity to control and maintain normal weight. Sixty minutes a day of moderately intense physical exercise is now recommended, doubling the daily minimum goal set by the 1996 Surgeon General's report. This new physical activity level is based on the amount of energy expended on average each day by persons who maintain a healthy weight. Walking 3.5 to 4 miles per hour, for a total of 60 minutes, or jogging 20 to 30 minutes, 5 to 7 days per week, or their equivalents, are considered sufficient physical exercise to accomplish this goal. The National Center for Chronic Disease Prevention and Health Promotion provides a key report on "Physical Activity and Good Nutrition: Essential Elements to Prevent Chronic Diseases" at: http://www.cdc.gov/nccdphp/aag/aag_dnpa.htm

The Economic Research Service (ERS) of the USDA provides continuing key food survey (CSFII) data on consumption of foods and nutrient intake and determines where dietary deficiencies, and over consumption, problems may exist. This report is available at: http://www.ers.usda.gov/briefing/DietandHealth/data

Dietary Reference Intakes (DRIs) have been established using an expanded concept that includes indicators of good health, prevention of chronic disease, and avoidance of adverse effects/toxicity due to over consumption. Thousands of studies reviewed by IOM/FNB link excessive, or inadequate consumption, of carbohydrates, fats, and proteins with increased risk for dietary deficiency diseases, diabetes, heart disease, obesity, and other chronic disorders. The new DRIs not only recommend proper dietary intakes intended to help individuals meet their daily nutritional requirements but also provide tolerable upper intake levels (ULs) that help them avoid potential harm from consuming too much.

DRIs are intended to meet the needs of persons who are essentially healthy and free of conditions that may alter their daily nutritional requirements. Individuals known to have specific disorders should obtain nutritional advice from their health care provider/physician, tailored to their special needs.

Adults should consume at least 130 grams of carbohydrates daily according to the latest guidelines. This level of intake is based on the minimum amount of carbohydrate required to produce enough glucose for the brain to function properly. Refined sugars added to the diet should compromise no more than 25% of total calories consumed.

Owing to the fact that saturated fat and cholesterol play no known beneficial health role, they are not required at any level in the diet. However, eliminating them entirely from the diet would be very difficult in terms of meeting other nutritional needs. Therefore, IOM/FNB recommends keeping consumption of them as low as feasible while maintaining a nutritionally adequate diet.

Monounsaturated and polyunsaturated fatty acids are also present in dietary fat. When they replace saturated fats in the diet, they lower the risk of cardiovascular disease. Two types of polyunsaturated fatty acids are essential and a lack of either one results in a deficiency state. The IOM/FNB report now sets recommended intake (RDAs) for linoleic acid (an omega-6 fatty acid) and alpha linolenic acid (an omega-3 fatty acid). Linoleic acid is present in high levels in vegetable oils such as safflower or corn oils, and alpha linolenic acid is found in milk and some vegetable oils such as soybean and flaxseed oils.

Partially hydrogenated vegetable oils, such as those used in many products, contain a particularly undesirable form of unsaturated fat known as trans fatty acids (TFAs). They have physical properties, and undesirable effects in the body, resembling saturated fatty acids, but worse. TFAs are present in many thousands of products such as stick (hard) margarine, shortenings, cookies, crackers, dairy products, meats, and fast foods. They are reported to increase the levels of "bad" cholesterol in blood, and the risk of cardiovascular disease, type 2 diabetes mellitus, and other chronic disorders. TFAs provide no known health benefit, and are not essential, therefore, no safe level of TFAs exists. Individuals should eat as little of them as feasible while consuming an otherwise nutritionally adequate diet.

Recommended intake levels for fiber also are provided in the IOM/FNB report based on studies that show an increased risk for cancer and cardiovascular disease when diets low in fiber are consumed. Fiber may be defined as the edible, undigestible complex carbohydrates and lignin naturally found in plant food. However, lack of a uniform acceptable definition of fiber for regulatory purposes casts doubt on the usefulness of some content claims of many new food products marketed as containing fiber.

Finally, for the first time requirements for all 9 essential amino acids found in dietary protein have been established, and the recommended intake of protein is reaffirmed.

1.2 Dietary Reference Intakes (DRIs)

IOM/FNB provide DRIs for all food nutrients and electrolytes (sodium, potassium, chloride and sulfate) as well as water and other components of food that may influence health and disease. In so doing, consideration is given to the levels of intake that are compatible with good nutrition throughout the life span that may decrease the risk of chronic disease. Findings and recommendations of IOM/FNB form the basis for appropriate dietary standards and guidelines.

It is now recognized that intakes higher than previously recommended in prior years, of some nutrients, are important for promoting good health and performance, and preventing chronic disease. Growth in food fortification with nutrients, and the increased use of dietary supplements has provided further evidence that information regarding Recommended Dietary Allowances alone does not provide appropriate guidelines for adequate nutrient intake. As a result, in 1995, DRIs for recommended nutrient intakes were established to include:

- Recommended Dietary Allowance (RDA) as the average daily dietary intake of a nutrient that is sufficient to meet the requirement of nearly all (97-98%) healthy persons.

- Adequate Intake (AI), similar to the previously used Estimated Safe and Adequate Daily Dietary Intake (ESADDI), is established when an RDA cannot be determined because of lack of sufficient data/evidence to do so.

  N.B.—thus, a nutrient has either a RDA or an AI based on observed intakes of the nutrient by a group of healthy persons.

- Tolerable Upper Intake Level (UL) as the highest daily intake of a nutrient that is likely to pose no significant risk of adverse effects/toxicity.

  N.B.—as intake above the UL increases, the risk of adverse effects/toxicity rises.

- Daily Value (DV) as the daily nutrient intake amount that may be used to help consumers and healthcare providers more effectively plan a healthy diet. DVs merely help individuals obtain a perspective on what may be considered overall daily dietary needs for particular nutrients.

Daily Reference Values (DRVs) have been established for the energy producing nutrients (carbohydrate, fat and protein) and are based on the number of calories consumed per day. For nutrition labeling purposes, 2,000 calories has been established as the reference point. DRVs for the energy producing nutrients and fiber are calculated as follows:

- total fat based on 30% of calories

- saturated fat based on 10% of calories

- carbohydrate based on 60% of calories

- protein based on 10% of calories

- fiber based on 11.5 grams per 1,000 calories

Thus, for example, an adult who consumes 2,000 calories per day would have a recommended intake of fat of 54 grams per day [0.30 x 2,000 = 600 calories divided by 9 (calories per gram of fat) = 54 grams].

DRVs for some nutrients represent the upper limit that is considered desirable because they are linked to certain chronic disease, e.g., fat, saturated fat, and cholesterol to cardiovascular disease, and sodium to high blood pressure. Therefore, DRVs for fats, protein, carbohydrate, sodium and potassium labeling appear as follows:

- total fat: less than 65 grams

- saturated fat: less than 20 grams

- cholesterol: less than 300 milligrams

- protein: 50 grams

- carbohydrate: 300 grams

- fiber: 25 grams

- sodium: less than 2,400 milligrams

- potassium: 3,500 milligrams

1.3 Essential Vitamins/Minerals DRIs

RDAs (AIs), ULs, and DVs for the essential vitamins and minerals are tabulated below.

Essential Vitamins

Vitamin	RDA(AI)	UL	DV
Biotin	300 µg/d(AI)	N.D.	300 µg/d
Choline	550 mg/d(AI)	3,500 mg/d	550 mg/d
Folate	400 µg/d	1,000 µg/d	400 µg/d
Niacin	20 mg/d	35 mg/d	20 mg/d
Pantothenic Acid	10 mg/d (AI)	ND	10 mg/d
Riboflavin	1.7 mg/d	200 mg/d	1.7 mg/d
Thiamine	1.5 mg/d	ND	1.5 mg/d
Vitamin A	3,000 IU (M)	10,000 IU	3,000 IU/d (M)
	2,300 IU (F)		2,300 IU/d (F)
Vitamin B-6	2 mg/d	100 mg/d	2 mg/d
Vitamin B-12	6 µg/d (AI)	1,000 µg/d	6 µg/d
Vitamin C	90 mg/d (M)	2,000 mg/d	90 mg/d (M)
	75 mg/d (F)		75 mg/d (F)
Vitamin D	400 IU/d	2,000 IU/d	400 IU/d
Vitamin E	30 IU/d (AI)	1100-1500 IU/d	30 IU/d
Vitamin K	80 µg/d (AI)	30,000 µg/d	80 µg/d

Essential Minerals

Mineral	RDA(AI)	UL	DV
Calcium	1000 mg/d	2,500 mg/d	1000 mg/d
Chromium	120 µg/d	ND	120 ug/d
Copper	2 mg/d	10 mg/d	2 mg/d
Iodine	150 µg/d	1,100 µg/d	150 µg/d
Iron	18 mg/d	45 mg/d	18 mg/d
Magnesium	400 mg/d	ND	400 mg/d
Manganese	2 mg/d	11 mg/d	2 mg/d
Molybdenum	75 µg/d (AI)	2,000 µg/d	75 µg/d
Phosphorous	1000 mg/d	4,000 mg/d	1,000 mg/d
Selenium	70 µg/d	400 ug/d	70 ug/d
Zinc	15 mg/d	40 mg/d	15 mg/d

Legend for Vitamins/Minerals table above
M = male, F = female
ND = not determined due to lack of sufficient evidence
µg = microgram, mg = milligram
UL = maximum level of daily nutrient intake likely to pose little or no risk of adverse effects. UL represents total intake from food, water, and supplements. ULs are not established for biotin, pantothenic acid, and thiamine. In the absence of ULs, extra caution is warranted in consuming levels above recommended intakes.
AI = Adequate intake where no RDA could be established due to insufficient data

Above information in table was constructed chiefly from data provided by:

- National Academy of Sciences, Institute of Medicine, Food and Nutrition Board

  http://www.iom.edu/IOM/IOMHOME.
  nsf/Pages/Food+and+Nutrition+Board

- USDA Food and Nutrition Information Center

  http://www.nal.usda.gov/fnic

- Vitamins and Minerals: How Much Do You Need

  http://www.mayoclinic.com

It may not be harmful for most, but not necessarily all adults, to consume up three times the Recommended Dietary Allowance (RDA), or DV levels of essential vitamins and minerals under a doctor's supervision. In fact, many people appear to regularly do so through the foods they eat and the supplements that they take.

Additional information on DVs and RDAs is available at:
http://www.fda.gov (use search site)
http://www.fda.gov/fdac/special/foodlabel/dvs.html

1.4 Energy Nutrients

Energy nutrients are carbohydrates, fats and proteins. They are discussed in sections 1.5-1.7 respectively.

In meeting the body's daily energy needs while minimizing the risk for chronic disease, IOM/FNB recommends that adults should obtain:

- 45 to 65% from carbohydrate

- 20 to 35 % from fat, and

- 10 to 35% from protein

The suggested caloric energy intake for most average, reasonably healthy, normal weight, adults males and females is estimated in the table below:

Calories Per Day

Category	Age in Years	Light Activity	Moderate Activity	Heavy Activity
Males	19-24	2,700	3,000	3,000
	29-50	3,000	3,200	4,000
	51 plus	2,300	2,300	--
Females	19-24	2,000	2,100	2,600
	29-50	2,200	2,300	2,800
	51 plus	1,900	1,900	--

Carbohydrate, protein, and fat can substitute for each other to some extent in terms of meeting the body's caloric energy needs. Therefore, the ranges employed in the diet should be regarded as flexible for daily dietary planning by individuals. In planning keep in mind that when individuals consume low levels of fat combined with high levels of carbohydrate, high density lipoprotein cholesterol (HDL-C, "good" variety) decreases. On the other hand, high fat diets can lead to increases in low density lipoprotein cholesterol (LDL-C, "bad" cholesterol), and obesity and its complications, such as cardiovascular disease, particularly when caloric intake is increased as well.

Ranges provided for carbohydrate, protein, and fat allow individuals to make healthy, realistic food choices based on their food preferences and needs. The diet chosen by an individual should be balanced with appropriate activity, and calories consumed should be commensurate with height, weight and gender for sedentary, moderately, and higher levels of physical activity. Adults should spend a total of at least one hour each day, 5-7 days/week, in moderately intense physical exercise as permitted by health.

1.5 Carbohydrates

Most foods contain carbohydrates which are compounds that include fibers, starches, and sugars. Carbohydrates are a necessary part of a healthy diet because they provide the energy needed for physical activity, and keep organs functioning properly. Refined carbohydrate (added sugars) in the diet should comprise no more than 25% of total calories consumed. In this regard, added sugars are defined as those incorporated into foods and beverages during production, and are to be distinguished from natural sugars such as lactose in milk and fructose in fruits. Major sources of added sugars in the diet include candy, soft drinks, fruit drinks, pastries and other sweets all of which tend also to lower intakes of essential nutrients in the diet.

The Daily Value for carbohydrates in nutritional labeling is 60% of total calories, or 300 grams/day for a 2,000 calorie diet. Adults should consume a minimum of 130 grams of carbohydrate each day, the estimated minimum needed to produce enough glucose for the brain, nervous system and other tissues/organs to function properly. Additional carbohydrate information is available at:
http://www.nutrition.org/nutinfo/content/carb.shtml

A Harvard School of Public Health report provides information on: carbohydrates and health, glycemic index, popular diets, high carbohydrate/very low fat diets (Dr. Ornish, Pritiken, and Food for Life), low carbohydrate/high protein diets (Zone, Dr. Atkins, and Protein Power Lifeplan) and is available at:
http://www.hsph.harvard.edu/nutritionsource/carbohydrates.html

1.6 Proteins

In spite of the progress made in other areas of nutrition, much less is known today about protein and health. For the first time, requirements for all 9 essential amino acids found in proteins have been determined. In addition, the previously established recommended levels of protein intake of 0.8 gram per kilogram (0.36 grams per pound) of body weight have been reconfirmed for men and women. This amount is needed for an adult to remain in nitrogen balance ("protein" balance) and to keep from slowly breaking down (catabolizing) their own tissues. Essential amino acid requirements are beyond the scope of this book and will not be discussed further.

Not all proteins are alike. Some contain all the essential amino acids needed to construct new proteins, and these are called complete proteins. Animal protein sources tend to be complete. Other proteins lack one or more essential amino acids, and are classified as incomplete (typically those found in fruits, vegetables, grains and nuts). Vegetarians and individuals who do not eat meat, fish, poultry, eggs or dairy products need to eat a variety of protein containing foods each day to avoid the health consequences of consuming only incomplete proteins.

Both too little and too much protein may result in serious health problems. Protein digestion/metabolism releases acids. The body neutralizes these acids, usually with calcium and other substances. High protein, low carbohydrate diets require a good deal of body calcium to neutralize acids formed, and the calcium used is made available from body stores, chiefly bone, leading to decalcification and increased susceptibility to fractures. For example, in the Nurses' Health Study, women who ate 95 grams of protein a day, were some 20% more likely to suffer a broken wrist over a 12 year period compared to those consuming less than 68 grams of protein a day.

In terms of health consequences, both animal and vegetable protein appear to produce similar effects in most instances. However, those protein sources with the highest amounts of saturated fat content appear to increase the risk of cardiovascular disease, stroke, and other age related disorders. Also red meats appear to increase the risk of colon cancer. Fish and poultry, on the other hand, are considered to be better alternatives to beef, and vegetable sources of protein may be even better.

Soy protein is a special case in terms of reducing chronic disease and promoting good health. Regularly consumed soy based foods are reported to lower blood cholesterol and triglycerides, reduce symptoms of menopause, prevent breast and prostrate cancer, promote weight loss, and decrease the risk of cardiovascular disease and osteoporosis. Beneficial effects of soy products may be due, at least in part, to their content of isoflavones, plant based phytoestrogens.

A ULs for protein has not been established because studies indicating the potential for high protein diets to produce chronic or other diseases are considered to be conflicting or inadequate to draw firm conclusions at this time,. However, caution is urged regarding any over consumption of protein and essential amino acids until this matter is clarified as recent research indicates that high protein intake may damage organ systems such as the kidneys.

A discussion of protein and its relationship to chronic disease is available at:
http://www.hsph.harvard.edu/nutritionsource/protein.html
http://www.nutrition.org/nutinfo/content/prot.shtml

1.7 Fats

Fats not only remain a major source of energy for the body but also aid in the absorption of nutrients such as the fat soluble vitamins. Margarine, vegetable oils, visible fat on meat and poultry, whole milk, egg yolks, and nuts are major contributors of fat in the diet. Saturated fats in high fat diets tend to raise low density lipoprotein cholesterol (LDL-C, or "bad" cholesterol) in blood and increase the risk of cardiovascular disease. The main sources for saturated fats in the diet include meats, baked goods and full fat dairy products. Saturated fats do not provide any known health benefits and therefore are not required in the diet. Thus, saturated fat intake should be kept low, e.g., less than 8% in an otherwise nutritionally adequate diet.

Monounsaturated (MUFAs) and polyunsaturated fatty acids (PUFAs) also are present in varying degrees in dietary fat. When they replace saturated fats in the diet, MUFAs and PUFAs tend to reduce total blood cholesterol levels, and LDL-C, and lower the risk of cardiovascular disease.

Individuals must obtain two types of PUFAs, alpha linolenic acid (ALA), an omega-3 fatty acid, and linoleic acid (LOA), an omega-6 fatty acid, from the diet since the body cannot make either and they are considered essential. Deficiency of either may result in scaly skin and dermatitis among other disorders. IOM/FNB recommended intakes for these two types of essential fatty acids to prevent deficiency states are:

• LOA = 17 grams/day for men, 12 grams/day for women

- ALA = 1.6 grams/day for men, 1.1 grams/day for women

See http://www.wadsworth.com/nutrition_d/special_features/breaking.html

A Harvard School of Public Health report describing the "good" and the "bad" fats, cholesterol, types of fats (in common oils, cooking fats, margarines/spreads), dietary fats (in relation to cardiovascular disease, cancer, and obesity), recommendations for fat intake and lowering trans fat consumption is available at:
http://www.hsph.harvard.edu/nutritionsource/fats.html

1.8 Trans Fats

1.8.1. Introduction

Partially hydrogenated unsaturated fatty acids, made from vegetable oils, are used in a number of margarines, shortenings, baked goods, and processed foods. These are called trans fatty acids (TFAs) and have physical properties resembling saturated fatty acids. Partially hydrogenated vegetable oils have been used extensively to replace tropical oils, beef tallow, and animal fats in processed foods because of lower cost, more functionality in product development, improved shelf life, and the fact that they do not contain cholesterol.

Until recently, health benefits regarding cholesterol have been claimed for stick (hard) margarine as a replacement for butter without regard for the trans fat content. The same held true for many other products containing partially hydrogenated oils and little or no cholesterol even though they contained high levels of TFAs.

Unsaturated fatty acids present in natural foods usually are in what is called the "cis" chemical configuration meaning that the hydrogen atoms are on the same side of the unsaturated double bond in the molecule. TFAs, produced by heating liquid unsaturated vegetable oils in the presence of metal catalysts and hydrogen in a process called partial hydrogenation, results in the hydrogen atoms being reconfigured on opposite sides of the double bond resulting in a more solid state trans fatty acid with a higher melting point. When trans fatty acids are ingested and incorporated into the walls of cells, they adversely affect/damage the cell's ability to function properly.

Evidence has been accumulated over the years regarding the adverse effects of TFAs in relation to their contribution to the 20th century epidemic of cardiovascular disease, type 2 diabetes mellitus, and other chronic disorders. TFAs have been shown to produce significantly greater increases in the "bad" or low density cholesterol (LDL-C) while decreasing the "good" or high density lipoprotein cholesterol (HDL-C), compared with saturated fatty acids, increasing the risk of cardiovascular and other chronic diseases.

Based on more recent information from the CSFII (Continuing Survey of Food Intake by Individuals), it is estimated that the average male takes in 7-8 grams, and the average female 5-6 grams of trans fats a day. The amount of TFAs consumed in the American diet is associated with an increase risk of over 100,000 premature coronary heart disease deaths annually in the United States alone. And, this adverse trans fat risk is regarded as much stronger than that produced by saturated fat. Thus trans fats appear to represent an even greater danger to health and longevity than saturated fats. It is estimated that a decrease in trans fatty acid intake to 3-4 grams or less a day could result in at least a 25% decrease in coronary heart disease deaths and a 40% decrease in non-insulin-dependent diabetes mellitus. For additional information see: http://sln.fi.edu/brain/nutrition/fats/transfats.html

Also individuals who are high consumers of trans fats are more than twice as likely to develop Alzheimer's disease. And, women who eat the most trans fats appear to have twice the risk of developing lymphoma. Thus, reducing trans fats in the diet may be a way to lower the risk not only of lymphoma (cancer of lymph glands) but also Alzheimer's disease.

1.8.2 Reducing Dietary Trans Fats

It has been concluded by experts in the field that a significant reduction of partially hydrogenated trans fats in the US diet and replacement with (unhydrogenated) natural vegetable oils could produce significant health benefits that would be greater than that which may occur with corresponding reductions in saturated fat intake alone.

The food industry in the United States is only recently beginning to respond to the trans fat problem. Trans fat free margarines that are low in saturated fats, are now available, but the marketplace still remains heavily oriented towards hydrogenated margarines high in trans fats. About one third of all trans fats consumed in the US still come from hydrogenated margarines, and the remainder from baked goods, fast foods, and other prepared/fabricated/processed foods such as french fries, potato chips, salad dressings, etc. It remains unlikely that significant "change for the better" will occur until stronger federal regulation is implemented in upcoming years, or pressure from the medical/healthcare professions and the public via legal action, etc. provide the necessary incentives for change.

Some 40-50,000 food products are now on the market that contain partially hydrogenated vegetable oils, and around three-quarters of these contain at least 0.5 grams or more of trans fats per serving. Products containing more than 0.5 grams TFAs per serving need to be drastically reduced in number or eliminated entirely from the marketplace as soon as possible to improve the health of the nation.

There are no known TFAs health benefits and they are considered potentially harmful to health. Also, the IOM/FNB have declared that there is no safe level (UL), and individuals should consume as little TFAs as feasible in an otherwise nutritionally adequate diet.

To help accomplish this goal individuals should:

- use naturally occurring, unhydrogenated oils such as canola or olive oil

- consume processed foods made with unhydrogenated oil rather than hydrogenated, or saturated fat

- choose soft (liquid or tube) margarine over harder, stick forms with no more than 2 grams of saturated fat per serving.

- cut back on snacks such as cookies, cakes, potato chips, tortilla chips, corn chips and other "junk foods", and substitute healthier snacks such as fresh or dried fruits, carrot sticks, and other vegetables, "no fat" pretzels, and air popped popcorn, or some trans fat free liquid spread

- reduce or eliminate home use or restaurant consumption of prepared and highly processed foods such as frozen, and deep fried foods (e.g. fried chicken, french fries, hash brown potatoes, potato puffs, fish sticks, tacos, or mozzarella sticks)

- eliminate or reduce intake of baked goods, remembering the rule, the sweeter the product, the more trans fats.

- limit daily intake of trans fats to less than 3-4 grams a day.

A cup of whole milk has around 0.3 grams of trans fats whereas a cup of low fat yogurt has only 0.1 gram of trans fat in comparison. Also, a 3.5 oz of turkey provides only around 0.05 grams trans fats in white meat and 0.15 grams in dark meat. All this should be compared with a doughnut with 3.5 to 4.0 grams of trans fats, potato chips with 3.0 grams per ounce, or a median order of french fries with around 7.5 grams. Most of the trans fats in the US diet come from foods such as stick margarine (3 grams trans fats per serving), and partially hydrogenated vegetable shortening (2.5 grams per serving).

A partial list of foods that are reasonably high in trans fats, and are to be avoided, or at least significantly reduced in the diet, include:

- beef
- beef fat (tallow)
- biscuit (KFC)*
- biscuit
- breakfast bar
- brownie
- butter
- cake
- candy bar
- cheese sandwich

- french fries
- frosting (creamy)
- granola bar
- hot dog (beef)
- lard
- margarine (stick)
- mayonnaise (regular)
- onion rings (fast food)
- pastry (Danish)
- pie

- cheesecake

- chicken dinner (KFC)*

- chicken nuggets

- cinnamon bun or roll

- cookies

- crackers

- doughnut

- fish sandwich (BK)**

- popcorn (microwave or butter/oil popped)

- salad dressing (ranch)

- scone (S)***

- shortening (Crisco or generic)

- shrimp (fried)

- taco shell

- tortilla chips

*KFC = Kentucky Fried Chicken
**BK = Burger King

***S = Starbuck's

1.8.3 Trans Fat Food Labeling

The FDA had proposed that trans fat content of foods be listed separately from saturated fats, and stating on the label that "intake of trans fats should be as low as possible". Such label wording was based on the IOM/FNB report indicating that available scientific evidence suggested that a safe, tolerable upper intake level (UL) of trans fats may approach zero. However, since trans fats are essentially unavoidable in most diets in the United States, achieving a UL of zero would require such extraordinary changes in dietary intake patterns that this effort might result in other unknown health risks. Therefore, a UL was not established, rather it was recommended that trans fat consumption be as low as possible while consuming a nutritionally adequate diet.

After about 10 years of debate, the FDA reached a settlement with the Food Industry in early 2003, and will require manufacturers' food nutrition labels to fully reveal the levels of trans fats directly on the label. A new line on the label will list the amount of trans fat under the amount of saturated fat. However, the new nutrition labels are not required to display the message that trans fat consumption should be as low as possible in their diet. Such a statement, originally proposed for inclusion in the label by the FDA, apparently had to be omitted due to objections voiced by the food industry. And, food companies still have until January 2006 to phase in the required, new trans fat content, nutrition label changes. This new trans fat labeling not only will help consumers reduce the deleterious levels of trans fat consumption in existence today, but also will provide a disincentive for the food industry to use partially hydrogenated oils (trans fats) in their products.

Until the trans fat nutrition labeling is put into place by manufacturers, individuals can estimate the trans fat content of a product by adding any monounsaturated, polyunsaturated, and saturated fat content and subtracting this combined amount from the total fat content on the label. This difference may then be regarded as a rough estimate of the trans fat content of a product serving.

Additional trans fat information is available at:
http://www.hsph.harvard.edu/reviews/transfats.html
http://sln.fi.edu/brain/nutrition/fats/transfats.html
http://www.ftc.gov/be/v030003.htm
http://www.healthcastle.com/trans_scam.shtml
http://www.fda.gov (search "trans fat")

1.9 Dietary Fiber

1.9.1 Introduction

The term fiber refers to complex carbohydrates found in the food that cannot be digested and assimilated and therefore provide no calories. Fiber is generally grouped into two broad categories according to the ease with which it dissolves in water. Soluble fiber dissolves, and insoluble fiber does not dissolve to any significant extent in water. This difference in solubility is regarded as important in terms of fiber's utility and health benefits.

Principal food sources for soluble fiber include apples, berries, legumes (beans, dried peas, and lentils), nuts, oat bran or oatmeal and pears. Insoluble fiber on the other hand, is found in such foods as carrots, celery, cucumbers, seeds, prunes, tomatoes, wheat bran, whole grains (barley, brown rice, bulgar, couscous), whole wheat bread, and whole grain breakfast cereals.

1.9.2 Recommended Fiber Intake

The IOM/FNB recently published a new daily recommended intake for fiber for adults. For men up to 50 years of age, intake should be 38 grams of fiber daily, for women, 25 grams daily. Men and women over 50 should consume 30 grams and 21 grams, respectively, of fiber daily. In order to increase fiber intake to these new levels, one should consider:

- whole grain cereals for breakfast

- whole fruits and vegetables instead of juices (unpeeled fruits and vegetables since much of the fiber is found in the skin)

- eating vegetables raw or steamed as other cooking methods may reduce fiber content

- consuming dried fruits as snacks

- brown rice and other whole grain products instead of white rice and refined grains and pasta, for meals

- raw vegetable snacks instead of chips, cookies, chocolate bars and crackers

- using legumes (beans, dried peas, and lentils) in chili and soups instead of meat

- fiber supplements as needed to meet recommended daily intake

See http://www.wadsworth.com/nutrition_d/special_features/breadking.html

1.9.3 Benefits of Dietary Fiber

Adequate fiber intake is regarded as an essential part of a healthy diet. It is reported to significantly reduce the risk of developing constipation, diabetes mellitus (non-insulin-dependent, type 2), diverticular disease, cardiovascular disease, and overweight and obesity, but not necessarily colon polyps or colon cancer. In fact, a large recent study provided reasonably good evidence that dietary fiber is not strongly associated with reduced risk for either colon cancer or polyps (a precursor to colon cancer). However, a recent large European clinical study has demonstrated the association of a reduced incidence of laryngeal cancer following dietary high fiber intake.

Constipation is one of the most common gastrointestinal complaints, particularly in the elderly. Consumption of adequate daily amounts of fiber not only relieves, but also may prevent, constipation. However, as fiber absorbs significant amounts of water, at least six 8 ounce glasses of water should be consumed each day to help optimize the beneficial effects of fiber in relieving or preventing constipation.

A diet high in whole grain cereal fiber has been linked positively to a lower risk of type 2 diabetes mellitus. In addition, a diet low in whole grain cereal fiber and high in high glycemic index foods (ones that increase blood sugar levels), adversely affects satisfactory control of blood sugar levels in diabetics. High fiber intake, on the other hand, helps to normalize blood sugar levels in diabetics. Low glycemic index/high fiber foods such as bran, legumes, whole fruits, and whole grain cereals also improve control of diabetic blood sugar levels. High glycemic index/low fiber foods such as potatoes, white bread, white rice, refined cereals, (e.g., corn flakes and Cherrios), white spaghetti, and refined carbohydrates tend to make control of blood sugar levels in diabetics more difficult.

Dietary fiber also is considered to be important in the prevention and treatment of diverticular disease, estimated to occur in 30-40% of individuals over the age of 50, and in three quarters of those over the age of 75. Eating a diet high in fiber is reported to lower the risk of diverticular disease by as much as 40%. High fiber diets/supplements also may be as useful in the treatment of irritable bowel syndrome.

High dietary fiber intake is reported to be associated with a 30-50% lower risk of cardiovascular disease. Whole grain cereal fiber may be particularly effective in this regard. Individuals with high cholesterol may also benefit from extra fiber in their diet. Individuals on cholesterol lowering drugs and a fiber rich diet may be able to lower their medication dosage, and even discontinue such medication in selected cases under the supervision of a physician.

Fiber rich foods also may help individuals lose weight and/or maintain weight loss because they are lower in calories, take longer to chew, tend to make one feel fuller faster and longer, and reduce daily fat consumption, a key to weight control. Adding two servings of a high fiber cereal per day to the diet (around 14 grams of fiber) is reported to reduce daily fat intake by about 10% and cholesterol by 20%.

In general, insoluble fiber is regarded as more likely to interfere with mineral absorption compared with soluble fiber. Also, substances such as phytates and oxalates found in grains, seeds, dried beans and some vegetables may decrease the absorption of calcium, iron and zinc. However, mineral deficiencies are unlikely if the diet comes from a variety of foods.

Evidence that long term use of fiber supplements such as Citrucel or Metamucil, or a high fiber diet may produce harmful effects is lacking. In fact, many doctors routinely recommend indefinite intake of high fiber diets and/or fiber supplements in patients with diverticular disease and irritable bowel syndrome and other disorders, and regard both as safe over the long term.

For regularity and constipation relief, insoluble fiber from wheat bran or whole grains, or a supplement such as Citrucel is considered to be useful. Oatmeal or other water soluble dietary fiber sources, or a supplement such as Metamucil (psyllium) may be considered to be more appropriate for controlling blood cholesterol or sugar levels.

Additional information on fiber and dietary food sources is available at:
http://www.hsph.harvard.edu/nutritionsource/fiber.html
http://www.nlm.nih.gov/medlineplus
http://www.mayoclinic.com
http://www.americanheart.org
Search "dietary fiber" on the last 3 websites.

1.10 Fish/Fish Oils

Fish are regarded as nutritious, healthful foods, rich in protein, low in carbohydrate, and packed with vitamins and minerals. Certain types of fish, especially the "fatty", cold-water varieties (i.e., sardines, salmon, herring, mackerel, halibut, stripped bass, tuna, and cod) are regarded as particularly healthful because of their rich content of omega-3 fatty acids (omega-3s), namely alpha linolenic acid (ALA), eicosapentanoic acid (EPA), and docosahexanoic acid (DHA). Humans cannot make these polyunsaturated fatty acids, and therefore they are considered essential and must be obtained from dietary sources, or from supplements.

Diet is regarded as the best source of omega-3s. Cold water fatty fish, great northern beans, kidney beans, navy beans and soybeans plus a variety of nuts are among the best dietary sources for omega-3s. Fish oil concentrates and flaxseed or flaxseed oils also are good supplement sources for omega-3s.

However, it is still unclear exactly how much fish/fish oil must be consumed daily to produce optimum health. Research indicates that 1-2 servings of fatty fish per week may suffice. Fatty fish are reported to have 10-15 times the omega-3 levels as lean fish. The average American may eat much less fish than recommended. Around 20% or more Americans eat no fish at all. One to two teaspoons of flaxseed or flaxseed oil, or 1-3 grams of fish oil omega-3s as a daily supplement provide ample intake under most circumstances.

The approximate level of omega 3s in various fish servings is given in the table below.

Fish	Serving size	Omega-3s
Salmon, Atlantic	6 oz	3-4 grams
Sardines, packed in oil	3 oz	3 grams
Salmon, coho	6 oz	2 grams
Herring, kippered	3 oz	2 grams
Trout, rainbow	6 oz	2 grams
Swordfish	6 oz	1.5 grams
Oysters	3 oz	1 gram
Mackerel	3 oz	1 gram
Sole or flounder	6 oz	1 gram

Stripped bass	6 oz	1 gram
Tuna, white, canned	3 oz	0.7 gram
Tuna, fresh	6 oz	0.5 gram

Clinical evidence suggests that fish/omega-3s may:

- reduce risk of cardiovascular disease, stroke, heart attacks, arrhythmias, and sudden death

- protect against breast, and endometrial cancer, and inhibit the growth of colon, pancreatic, and prostate cancers

- prevent cachexia (wasting/malnourishment) occurring in the late stages of some cancers

- be useful in the treatment of arthritis, depression, migraine headaches and possibly bipolar disorder and schizophrenia.

The Lyon Heart Study, demonstrated that a diet high in alpha linolenic acid (omega-3s) and low in linoleic acid (omega-6s) was associated with a 47% reduction in cardiac events, a 76% reduction in major events, and a 56% lower risk of dying during the 4 year study period.

The US DART trial demonstrated that eating just two portions of fish per week reduces the risk of a heart attack and sudden death by 29% in patients with coronary heart disease.

In an Italian study of some 11,000 heart attack survivors, researchers found that those taking a daily fish oil capsule (containing omega-3 fatty acids) were 42% less likely to suffer a second heart attack or die compared with those not taking the supplement

In another study of 16,000 Italians, those who ate fish twice a week had half the risk of cancer of the rectum and oral cavity, and lower risks of cancer of the esophagus, stomach, colon, and pancreas compared to those who ate fish less than once a week

A 5,000 Dutch patient study demonstrated that individuals (average age 67) who ate at least 4 ounces of fish a week (1 serving) were 70% less likely to develop Alzheimer's disease over a two year period.

Men with the highest levels of omega-3s in their blood are reported to be more than 80% less likely to die suddenly from heart disease. However, it should be recognized that eating more than the recommended amount of fish per week appears to offer no additional protection in this regard. In fact, most studies show that eating 1-2 servings of "fatty" fish per week significantly lessens one's chance of a heart attack.

The American Heart Association (AHA) recommends at least 2 servings of fish (preferably the "fatty" kind) per week. Omega-3s seem to be particularly protective against sudden cardiac arrest and death which account for around 50% of the half million cardiac deaths in the United States each year, principally caused by arrhythmias (omega-3s appear to "stabilize heart cells electrically").

Additionally, omega-3s are reported to help prevent endometrial and prostrate cancers presumably by reducing the levels of certain tumor promoting prostaglandins. Omega-3s have been reported to actually kill human breast cancer cells in tissue culture.

Omega-3s also appear to aid in neural development and help modulate the function of neurotransmitters in the brain which may account, at least in part, for their reported usefulness in depression, migraine headaches, and bipolar disorders.

While a number of claims for health benefits have been made for omega-3s, far more clinical research is still needed to fully establish their role in health as well as in the prevention/treatment of various disease states.

Mercury occurs naturally in small amounts in the environment, but has reached higher levels in the lakes, rivers and along the shorelines of populated areas due to pollution. Concentrations of mercury are high in some fish particularly the "fatty" ones and those larger ones that are higher up on the food chain. People who frequently eat fish they may catch in polluted areas may be more exposed to excessive mercury as well as other toxic pollutants. The Environmental Protection Agency indicates that US consumers eating most commercial fish generally are not exposed to such harmful effects in any known way. Therefore, health benefits from eating fish appear to outweigh the risks although concern exists for fetuses because even low levels of mercury or other pollutants may produce harmful effects in them. For most others, however, the bottom line on fish consumption appears to be that when fish come from a reliable, well regulated commercial source, eating fish, in moderate amounts 1-2 times a week, likely still deserves a healthy reputation.

However, it is recommended that one should:

- avoid shark, swordfish, king mackerel, and tile fish which appear to have the highest levels of mercury exceeding the FDA's advisory limit of one part per million,

- restrict walleye, pike, bass, muskie, and other freshwater fish to 2-3 ounces or one meal per week,

- restrict to 2-3 meals per week fish such as canned tuna, shrimp, pollock, salmon, cod, catfish, clams, flounder, halibut, sole, crabs, and scallops, all of which account for about 85% of the fish we eat, and have low enough mercury levels so that a couple of meals per week may be considered safe.

Additional research has focused on the role of omega-3s in relation to omega-6s fatty acids found in many vegetable oils, cereals, snack foods and baked goods. An imbalance in the ratio of omega-3s to omega-6s may play a role in the development of cancer and other chronic diseases. The typical American diet is reported to be low in omega-3s and high in omega-6s (10 to 20 times more), and women with breast cancer have 2 to 5 times more omega-6s in their bodies, suggesting that an abnormal ratio of 3s to 6s may play a role in breast cancer.

Additional information regarding fish/fish oil is available via search sites at:
http://www.americanheart.org
http://www.cancer.gov
http://www.nlm.nih.gov/medlineplus
http://www.fda.gov

A report entitled "Mercury in Fish: Cause for Concern" is available at:
http://www.fda.gov/fdac/reprints/mercury.html

1.11 Flaxseed/Flaxseed Oils

Flaxseed is not only high in fiber but also in omega-3 essential fatty acids. It is the richest plant source of alpha linolenic acid (ALA), a principal omega-3 fatty acid. While fish oil contains two key omega-3 fatty acids, eicosapentanoic (EPA) and docosahexanoic (DHA), flaxseed is rich principally in ALA, a key precursor to both EPA and DHA. The body converts ALA into EPA and somewhat more slowly into DHA. Approximately 10-12 grams of ALA are needed to convert to around 1 gram of EPA and DHA in the body. However, it should be noted that diets rich in trans fatty acids decrease the conversion of ALA into EPA and DHA in the body.

Linoleic acid is the primary omega-6 fatty acid in flaxseed oil. It is converted in the body principally to gamma linolenic acid (GLA) and subsequently to EPA/DHA.

A diet rich in flaxseed is reported to decrease size, aggressiveness, and severity of prostate tumors in mice. In men with prostate cancer, flaxseed added to the diet may decrease testosterone as well as PSA (prostate specific antigen) levels in blood. Flaxseed in the diet also is reported to significantly reduce breast and colon tumors in animals, and decrease the risk of heart disease and stroke. Lignans (phytoestrogens) in flaxseed may be responsible for some of these effects. Processing flaxseed to flaxseed oils removes the potentially beneficial lignans.

Omega-6 to omega-3 imbalance in the diet appears to be linked with increased risk of cardiovascular disease, cancer, insulin resistance/diabetes mellitus, immune disorders (e.g., lupus), schizophrenia, depression, accelerated aging, stroke, obesity, arthritis, and Alzheimer's disease. The risk for such diseases appears to be least when no more than 2-4 times as much omega-6 compared with omega-3 is consumed daily in the diet. Unfortunately, Americans tend to consume some 10 to 30 times more omega-6s than omega-3s, putting them at significant risk for serious and disabling chronic disease.

Flaxseed may be used as a dietary supplement for its high fiber content as well as for a source of essential fatty acids to meet dietary requirements. Flaxseed oils also may provide an important source for dietary essential fatty acid intake, different from, and complimenting, fish/fish oils in the diet.

Additional flaxseed/oil information is available at:
http://www.sciencedaily.com/releases/2001/07/010712080024.htm

The full text of the National Academy of Sciences DRIs for energy, carbohydrate, fiber, fat, fatty acids, cholesterol, protein and amino acids is available at:
http://ww.nap.edu

An abbreviated outline of the content of the above NAS report is available at:
http://www.wadsworth.com/nutrition_d/special_features/breaking.html

2. Dietary Guidelines for Americans

2.1 Introduction

The Food and Nutrition Information Center (FNIC) is part of the US Department of Agriculture (USDA) and the Agricultural Research Service (ARS). It has a Cooperative Agreement with the University of Maryland's Department of Nutrition. FNIC provides state-of-the-art information and has issued "Dietary Guidelines for Americans" which is available at: http://www.nal.usda.gov/fnic/dga/index.html

Information about nutrition topics A-Z, dietary supplements, food composition, dietary guidelines, and the food guide pyramid also may be found at: http://www.nal.usda/fnic

2.2 ABCs of Dietary Guidelines

The ABCs of Dietary Guidelines for Americans include the following broad principals:

- Aim for fitness
  - aim for a healthy weight/energy balance
  - be physically active each day

- Build a healthy nutritional base
  - let the Pyramid guide your food choices
  - eat a variety of grains daily, especially whole grains
  - consume a variety of fruits and vegetables daily
  - keep food safe to eat
- Choose a sensible diet
  - low in saturated fat and cholesterol, moderate in total fat and low in transfat
  - moderate/reduce intake of refined sugars in beverages and foods
  - eat foods low in salt
  - use alcohol in moderation, or not at all

2.3 Aim for fitness

In order to aim for fitness, individuals need to choose a lifestyle that combines sensible eating with regular physical activity. Individuals need to avoid gaining weight, and maintain normal weight/energy balance. Being overweight or obese increases the risk for complications of chronic diseases such as arthritis, breathing problems, certain types of cancer, diabetes mellitus (non-insulin-dependent type 2), heart disease, high blood pressure, and stroke. A healthy weight, sound nutrition, and exercise provide key ways to help avoid chronic diseases and to live a longer, healthier life. In addition to being active whenever feasible, adults should engage in moderate physical exercise, for 60 minutes each day, as permitted by health status.

Different methods are used to determine if body weight may be considered normal or otherwise. One commonly used method is the estimate of Body Mass Index (BMI), a measure that determines if weight is "about right for height".

An expert panel, convened by the National Institute of Health in 1998, recommended that BMI be used to classify normal weight, overweight and obesity because it:

- correlates well with total body fat for the majority of people, and with the risk of disease complications and death

- is easily calculated "by hand" or with a calculator as follows:

  BMI = weight in pounds divided by height in inches squared, times 703

A BMI calculator is available at:
http://www.cdc.gov/nccdphp/dnpa/bmi/calc-bmi.htm

The relationship between BMI and disease risk is summarized in the table below:

Classification	BMI	Disease Risk*
Normal weight	18.5-24.9	normal
Overweight	25.0-29.9	low
Obesity		
• Mild, Class I	30.0-34.9	moderate
• Moderate, Class II	35.0-39.9	high
• Severe, Class III	>40	very high

*for serious disease complications such as diabetes mellitus, high blood pressure, heart disease, stroke, etc.

Classification by BMI and disease risk information is available at:
http://www.nhlbi.nih.gov/health/public/heart/obestiy/lose_wt/bmi_dis.htm

Additional information on physical activity and its benefits is available at:

- Nutrition and Physical Activity

  http://www.cdc.gov/nccdphp/dnpa/physcial/recommendations.htm

- Physical Activity Evaluation Handbook

  http://www.cdc.gov/nccdphp/dnpa/physical/handbook/index.htm

2.4 Build A Healthy Base/Food Guide Pyramid

No single food can supply all the nutrients, calories for energy, essential vitamins and minerals, phytochemicals, and other healthful substances in the amounts needed for optimum health. It is recommended by the Center for Nutrition Policy and Promotion that the Food Guide Pyramid be used as a starting point, choosing daily servings from each of the major food groups. If for any reason, certain foods from any of the five groups need to be avoided it is recommended that professional guidance be sought from a doctor.

Note that the number of servings needed from each of the 5 food groups depends on age. Serving size also is important. Plant foods (grains, fruits, and vegetables) at the base of the pyramid provide the foundation for meals. Individuals are encouraged to consume a variety of grains (especially whole grain foods), fruits and vegetables. A moderate amount of low fat foods from the milk, meat and beans groups may be included in meals. Reduce or avoid food high in fats, especially saturated and trans fats, or refined sugars and added salt.

Other principles considered to be important in a healthy diet include:

- limit intake of fats and oils

- choose vegetable oils rather than solid fats found in meats, dairy products, shortenings and stick (hard) margarine

- eat fish, shellfish, lean poultry, and lean meats, or nuts

- trim fat from meat and remove skin from poultry

- consume dry beans, peas or lentils more often

- avoid, or reduce, intake of liver and other organ meats as well as high fat processed meats (such as bacon, sausages, salami, bologna, and other cold cuts)

- use egg yolks in moderation and substitute egg whites when feasible

- select fat free or low fat milk, yogurt, and cheese

- check the nutrition label on prepared foods and choose those products lower in saturated fats, trans fats, and cholesterol

- in restaurants and other eating establishments,
    - choose fish or lean meats
    - limit or avoid ground and fatty processed meats, marbled steaks and cheese
    - avoid foods with creamy sauces
    - add little or no butter, mayonnaise, or margarine to food
    - choose fruits as desserts
    - beware of large serving sizes and consider taking home around half the restaurant meal for eating the next day.

Instructions on how to use the Food Guide Pyramid wisely are available at: http://www.pueblo.gsa.gov/cic_text/food/usingdietguide/cover.htm

Additional information on the Food Guide Pyramid and a healthy diet are available from the Center for Nutrition Policy and Promotion at: http://www.usda.gov/cnpp

2.5 Choose a Sensible Diet

Different individuals like different foods and even prefer preparing the same foods in different ways. Availability of food, allergies, culture, cost, family background, food intolerances, life experiences, moral beliefs, religion, and other factors may affect an individual's food choices. The Food Guide Pyramid allows individuals to make their choices from each of the major food groups and combine, cook, and eat them, as desired, taking into account their individual preferences while remaining within the dietary guidelines.

Literally thousands of different diets have been proposed over the years for a variety of reasons, mostly to control weight. Most are either beyond the scope of this book, or not recommended. A comparison of some of the more recent popularized diets can be found at:
http://www.dietsurf.com (click on "quickdietcomparisons")

Of the popularized diets, the Mediterranean and Pritikin diets may be suitable for many adults who are in reasonably good health. The "Mediterranean Diet" is discussed further in section 2.6. The Pritikin Diet may be found at:
http://www.dietsurf.com/diet/pritikin_diet.htm.

The Pritikin diet will not be discussed further. However, a similar one the Dr. Ornish Diet, is discussed under section 2.9.

The Mediterranean, Pritikin and Dr. Ornish diets may be considered reasonably sensible dietary choices for at least some otherwise healthy adults. However, both the Pritikin and Dr. Ornish diets are considered to be somewhat difficult for many people to follow long term.

For good nutritional health and a longer life, the USDA recommends choosing a sensible diet which includes:

- a variety of foods

- balance in the amount of food you eat with physical activity to control weight

- plenty of whole grain products, fruits, and vegetables

- low total fat, saturated fat, trans fats and cholesterol

- low to moderate sugar content

- moderate amounts of salt, sodium, and alcohol

The diet chosen should have most calories from whole grain foods, fruits, vegetables, low fat milk/products, lean meats, fish, poultry, dry beans, and fewer calories from fats, especially saturated and trans fats, as well as sweets. Bear in mind that:

- foods contain not only energy nutrients but other components that affect health

- physical activity fosters a more healthful diet

- a healthful diet contains the amounts of essential nutrients and calories needed to prevent nutritional deficiencies and excesses

- RDAs/DVs represent the amounts of nutrients that are adequate to meet the needs of most healthy people

- dietary guidelines describe food choices that promote good health

- food labels and the Food Guide Pyramid are tools to help you make intelligent food choices

In choosing a sensible diet, individuals should:

- follow healthy eating tips, start the day off right and eat breakfast

- drink 100% fruit juice with breakfast, or take a can to drink at work

- spruce up breakfast with a banana or a handful of berries with cereal, yogurt, waffles, or pancakes

- take a piece of fruit to munch during commute or work break

- when shopping, go to the produce section first for fruits and vegetables, and buy them. Keep bowls of fruit on the kitchen table and counter for a daytime snack.

- use butter and margarine sparingly. Switch to reduced fat or trans fat free margarine, or use fruit preserves on your whole grain bread toast. Limit your intake of baked goods to reduce harmful saturated and trans fat intake.

- consume "lite" or low fat dairy products (e.g., milk, cheese, yogurt, or sour cream).

- coat salads with low fat salad dressing.

- use light or fat free mayonnaise preferentially.

- choose the leanest cuts of meat, turkey, chicken breasts and roasts. Cuts with the name "loin" or "round" are leaner. Trim all visible fat before cooking meats, and drain the grease. Remove the skin from chicken.

- eat fried foods sparingly, if at all.

- substitute a baked potato for french fries.

- make healthier snacks, using celery sticks, cucumber wedges and cherry tomatoes.

- cut down on desserts and sweets, meal portion size, the number of full meals and choose mini meals more often.

- substitute low fat or fat free baked goods, cookies and ice cream for full fat products.

- choose fruit for dessert that is filling and provides energy

- remember that just because something is fat free or low fat, doesn't mean one can eat as much as wanted. Many low fat or nonfat foods also are high in calories, so eat everything in moderation.

- when eating out in a restaurant, eat half the meal and ask for the other half to take home in a "doggy bag". Remember, typical restaurant servings are often twice or more the size of a single serving.

- fast food restaurants cater to two of our favorite desires, "food" and "in a hurry". Unfortunately, much fast food also combines a lot of saturated, trans fats, and calories. Reduce the fat and calories by:
  - ordering a lean roast beef or grilled chicken sandwich
  - choosing more nutritious toppings
  - eliminating high fat dressings and cheese
  - keeping the portions regular and small

"Nutrition: Tips for Improving Your Health" is available at:
http://www.familydoctor.org/handouts/369.html

"Food Choice Recommendations for Reducing Cancer Risk" is available at: http://www.familydoctor.org/handouts/301.html

Information on "Healthy Eating Tips" is available at: http://www.calc.gov/nccdphp/dnpa/heal_eat.htm

Additional information for selecting a sensible diet is available at:
http://www.nal.usda.gov/fnic/dga
http://www.nal.usda.gov/fnic/dga/grains.htm

2.6 Mediterranean Diet/Pyramid

There are many different Mediterranean diets depending on which of the countries or localities on the Mediterranean Sea one chooses. Differences in agriculture, culture, economy, ethnic background, region, religion, and other factors results in diets that vary significantly among countries and regions. Nevertheless, a common basic Mediterranean dietary pattern emerges from all of this that is characterized principally by:

- a high intake of fruits and vegetables, whole grain breads and cereals, potatoes, beans, nuts and seeds

- preference for dairy products, fish and poultry as opposed to red meat

- use of olive oil as an important monosaturated fat source

- ingestion of eggs sparingly, zero to four times a week

- low to moderate intake of wine.

Generally, Mediterranean diets contain a relatively high percentage of calories from fat, and 40% or more of these fat calories come from monounsaturated fats (mostly olive oil). Monounsaturated fats are less effective is raising blood cholesterol/fat levels compared with the saturated fats. While the incidence of heart disease and the death rate in Mediterranean countries is reported to be lower than in the United States, this is not likely to be due solely to diet. Lifestyle factors and social structure, as well as other factors are believed to play a role as well.

Harvard researchers who monitored 22,000 Mediterranean individuals, found that those consuming the "classic Greek diet", one that is rich in olive oil, unrefined whole grains, high in fruits and vegetables, and accompanied by a moderate amount of wine, lived longer than those who did not. Among those who followed the diet most closely, the risk of death from heart disease was found to be 33% lower and the risk of death from cancer 24% lower.

In another study in 600 French men, a modified Mediterranean diet is reported to have produced nearly 70% fewer heart attacks and cardiac deaths. In this study, margarine, made by an esterification process, was used in place of butter. The esterification process results in a margarine without harmful trans fatty acids.

Research also suggests that a Mediterranean diet may ease the symptoms of rheumatoid arthritis, decreasing pain, inflammation, disease activity, and the number of swollen joints. Current results suggest that patients with rheumatoid arthritis may obtain better joint function as well as increased vitality from eating a Mediterranean diet.

Other research suggests that followers of a Mediterranean diet enjoy a wide range of health benefits such as a lower risk of cardiovascular disease, cancer, and memory loss with aging.

Individuals are cautioned that the high fat content of the Mediterranean diet may increase the risk of obesity and its health complications. More needs to be known about an optimal Mediterranean diet before it can be widely recommended especially for peoples from non Mediterranean countries.

Additional information on the Mediterranean diet is available at:
http://www.dietsurf.com/diet/mediterranean_diet.htm
http://www.nlm.nih.gov/medlineplus (search "Mediterranean diet")

2.7 AHA Dietary Guidelines

American Heart Association Dietary Guidelines recommend that individuals:

- balance levels of caloric intake and physical activity/exercise to control weight

- eat a nutritionally balanced diet consisting of a variety of foods

- eat 5 or more servings per day of a variety of fruits and vegetables

- consume 6 or more servings per day of a variety of grains, principally whole grains

- limit intake of food high in saturated fat, trans fat, cholesterol, and/or calories, or low in nutrition such as soft drinks, and candy/snacks high in refined sugar

- eat at least two servings of fish per week

- consume no more than 2400 milligrams of sodium per day

- drink no more than 1 to 2 ounces of alcohol per day.

Ample clinical evidence exists to support ability of individuals to comply, usefulness, and safety of these AHA guidelines, especially in individuals who are at risk for, or suffer from, cardiovascular disease, both in terms of prevention or treatment.

Additional information on AHA dietary guidelines is available at: http://www.americanheart.org (search "dietary guidelines")

2.8 Dr. Atkins Diet

The so-called "diet-revolution" championed by the late Dr. Robert C. Atkins has stirred up controversy over which diet is best for Americans to control their weight, or lose weight when needed. This diet was not designed to limit caloric intake or the amount of fat from meat, eggs, cheese, etc. consumed. It is based on the premise that high fat foods not only digest more slowly but they also make one feel satisfied longer, thus limiting food intake. Being low in carbohydrates, the Atkins diet causes the body to burn fat and manufacture ketones that suppress hunger further reportedly making it easier to adhere to over time. In addition, this diet may spare muscle loss and decrease blood glucose and insulin levels.

The Atkins diet is reported to be easier to follow and adhere to, and reasonably effective in maintaining normal weight. However, long term effectiveness and safety remain to be demonstrated in large scale well controlled clinical trials. On the negative side, there appears to be an increased risk of cardiovascular disease from the saturated fat content of the diet. Furthermore, the typical Atkins diet may be lacking in B vitamins and vitamins A, C and D, as well as antioxidants, phytonutrients, and calcium. Too much animal protein may lead to leaching of calcium from bone, increasing the risk of osteopenia, osteoporosis and fractures. As a result, patients on the Atkins diet usually require supplements of nutrients to avoid deficiencies.

Current interest in the Atkins diet appears to be due to claims that low to moderate fat diets may be more difficult to adhere to, or not work as effectively in weight control. However, such claims have not been demonstrated to be true in clinical trials to date. While the Atkins diet cannot be recommended at this time, additional information/details for those interested is available at:
http://www.Atkinscenter.com

2.9 Dr. Ornish Diet

The Dr. Ornish diet is at the other extreme of the diet controversy. With this diet, it is reported that you can "eat all you want", providing foods consumed are very low in fat and high in fiber. The fiber content is designed to fill one up, reduce hunger/desire to eat, and thus curtail food/calorie intake, and maintain normal weight.

Available evidence appears to indicate that the longer one follows such a very low fat, whole foods diet (complex carbohydrates such as unrefined whole grain bread, brown rice, fruits, vegetables, beans, etc.), the healthier one apparently becomes.

While Dr. Ornish's diet was originally designed mainly for people with cardiovascular disease, some of whom apparently were able to reverse the course of their disease for the better, this diet is now also considered useful for maintenance of normal weight, and prevention of overweight, obesity and health related complications.

Dr. Ornish's diet is not considered easy for most people to adhere to. Whether it eventually will prove acceptable to larger numbers of Americans remains to be seen. In the meantime, it may be considered in those for whom it may be appropriate, under a doctor's supervision.

Long term comparative well controlled clinical trials are needed to document compliance, usefulness and safety of the Dr. Ornish diet.

Additional information/details are available at:
http://www.ornish.com

2.10 Moderate Fat Diet

In the past, a diet of 30% total fat with less than 10% saturated fat was considered a low fat diet recommended by the US Dietary Guidelines for Americans, American Heart Association, and National Cholesterol Guidelines for NHLBI (National Heart, Lung and Blood Institute). Today, essentially the same diet is called a Moderate Fat Diet (MFD), and fat content may range from 20-30% of total calories consumed.

In contrast to the lack of substantial long term clinical trial evidence for the Atkins, Ornish, and Mediterranean diets, there are a number of such trials demonstrating not only compliance, utility, and safety of the MFD but also that reducing dietary fat is a practical way to decrease calories in the diet and promote weight control. Thus a MFD is one that appears to be sensible for most otherwise reasonably healthy individuals.

A MFD may include the following:

Calories	2,000 calories (1)
Total fat	20-30% of total calories (2)
Saturated fat	less than 8% of total calories
Monounsaturated fat	up to 8-10% of total calories
Polyunsaturated fat	up to 8-10% of total calories
Trans fat	less than 3-4 grams per day

Cholesterol	less than 300 mg/day
Carbohydrate	55% of total calories (3)
Protein	15% of total calories
Fiber	at least 25-30 grams/day (4)

1. caloric intake table adjusted according to gender, height and weight, and activity level for achieving and maintaining normal weight

2. derived from lean meat, fish and bean/plant sources

3. mainly complex carbohydrates from a variety of fruits, vegetables and whole grains, consisting of five to nine servings of fruits and vegetables per day

4. from food sources and/or supplements

Content needs to be in accordance with Dietary Guidelines for Americans. Fluid intake, in addition to that from foods consumed, should be in the order of 1.5 to 2.0 quarts of fluid (or its equivalent) daily. Vitamin and mineral intake should be supplemented as needed.

Additional information on dietary guidelines may be found at:
http://www.health.gov/dietaryguidelines

3. Phytonutients/Phytochemicals

3.1 Introduction

In addition to carbohydrate, fat, protein, fiber and essential vitamins and minerals, plant foods contain important substances collectively known as phytonutrients/phytochemicals that are regarded as disease preventive substances. Phyto is a prefix derived from the Greek word for plant, and phytonutrients are found in all plant foods. Phytonutrients give plants their odor, color, and flavor and help protect them from pests, viruses, bacteria, fungi, and excessive sunlight.

The study of phytonutrients and human health is a relatively new field of endeavor. Before any definitive recommendations can be made as to specific types and amounts of phytonutrients that may be regarded as beneficial to human health, and in what ways, much more research is needed. However, a significant amount of information now is available and some even consider phytonutrients as "Phytochemicals: Vitamins of the Future", and "Phytochemicals: Guardians of Our Health". These reports are available respectively at:

http://ohioline.osu.edu/hyg-fact/5000/5050.html
http://ww.andrews.edu/NUFS/phyto.html

Additional information is available at:
http://www.nutrition.org/nutinfo/content/phyt.shtml

Scientists appear to agree, from what is presently known, that phytonutrients generally do not act alone but rather do so synergistically as they coexist naturally with other nutrients/substances that may give them their unique qualities. Therefore, most agree that the best way to obtain potential benefits of phytonutrients is by eating a wide variety of plant foods, especially fruits and vegetables, whole grains, nuts and seeds.

In order to optimize the phytonutrient activity of foods, essentially the same storage, handling, and cooking recommendations for retaining vitamins in foods should be followed. Fresh fruits and vegetables should be obtained and consumed in season. Peeling needs to be limited as some phytonutrients are concentrated in the skins. Vegetables should be steamed, broiled or microwaved, using minimal amounts of cooking liquid to preserve water soluble phytonutrients.

A number of phytonutrients act as antioxidants and prevent free radical attack of cell membranes and damage to DNA. Free radicals are unstable molecules in the body resulting from normal metabolic processes such as activity/exercise, breathing, and digestion. During free radical production, molecules lose an electron which makes them unstable and they seek to restore stability by replacing the lost electron. They capture electrons from other molecules in the cell, mostly from cell membranes, damaging DNA, proteins, and lipids in the cell. This process begins a chemical chain reaction that produces even more free radicals. Free radicals also can be caused by ultraviolet light, x-rays, heat or pollutants.

Cells injured by free radicals may fail to activate their natural disease fighting defenses. Cellular damage may accumulate and result in a chronic disease. Available research implicates free radicals in a number of chronic degenerative disorders such as Alzheimer's, cancer, cardiovascular disease, cataracts, immune dysfunction, and age related macular degeneration. Antioxidants can donate electrons to these disease causing free radicals and stop them from damaging cells. They stabilize free radicals similar to the way coating apple slices with vitamin C/orange juice prevents browning.

Additional information on phytonutrients is available at:

- "Antioxidants and Cancer Prevention"

  http://www.cancer.gov

- "Antioxidants, Phytochemicals and Functional Foods"

  http://www.nal.usda.gov/fnic/consumersite/hot-antioxidants.htm

- "Phytochemicals: Nutrients of the Future"

  http://www.realtime.net/anr/phytonu.html

- Frequently asked questions/answers about phytonutrients/phytochemicals

  http://www.barc.usda.gov/bhnrc/pl/pl_faq.html

More specific information on any given phytonutrient/phytochemical of interest may be obtained by searching the Web resources provided in Chapter 7.

3.2 Disease Prevention Mechanisms

Based on available scientific evidence, a number of disease preventive mechanisms have been offered for consideration. Phytonutrients may:

- act as antioxidants

- aid in cell-to-cell communication

- alter hormone receptor binding

- block specific enzyme systems such as the angiotension converting enzyme (ACE) involved in raising blood pressure, or cyclooxygenase enzyme system involved in platelet stickness/clumping and the clotting of blood

- produce cancer cell death (apoptosis)

- detoxify carcinogens (via activation of cytochrome P450 and other enzyme systems)

- enhance immune responses

- convert precursors to active substances (e.g. alpha and beta carotene to vitamin A)

- modify gene expression by turning oncogene and tumor suppressor genes on or off

- repair DNA damage (e.g. due to smoking, pollution, or other toxic substance exposure such as alcohol)

The specific disease preventive mechanisms for any given phytonutrient or combination of phytonutirents that may be involved in any disease remain to be clarified.

3.3 Potential Health Benefits

A number of phytonutrients have been identified as having health benefiting properties. For example, phytonutrients are associated with the prevention and/or treatment of four of the leading causes of death in the United States, namely: cancer, cardiovascular disease, diabetes mellitus (non-insulin-dependent type 2), and hypertension, as well as other conditions such as cataracts and age related macular degeneration, the leading causes of blindness in the elderly.

Available research indicates that many forms of cancer are largely avoidable diseases, and more than two thirds may be prevented through lifestyle modification. It is estimated that around one third of these preventable cancers can be attributed to poor diet alone.

Consumption of fruits and vegetables has been consistently shown to reduce the risk of many cancers, and has led to the National Cancer Institute major prevention strategy of "5 to 9 a Day for Better Health", encouraging the public to include more fruits and vegetables in their diets.

In addition, the American Cancer Society guidelines for good nutrition and cancer prevention now include recommendations for:

- choosing most of the foods eaten from plant sources

- limiting intake of alcoholic beverages and high fat foods, particularly from animal sources

- being physically active and maintaining a healthy normal weight.

The recommendation "choose most of the foods you eat from plant sources" has been recognized for some time now as key for good nutrition and health.

Dietary Guidelines for Americans and the Food Guide Pyramid both recognize, emphasize, and illustrate this key recommendation. And, research studies have now identified specific phytochemicals in fruits, vegetables, grains, legumes, seeds, soy and tea that are being increasingly recognized for their potential in terms of protection against cancer, diabetes mellitus, cardiovascular diseases, cataracts, and age related macular degeneration as well as other chronic conditions.

To obtain additional phytonutrients in the diet, it is important for individuals to consume more whole grains, fruits, vegetables, seeds and nuts. An average American is reported to consume less than one serving of fruit and about one and one half serving of vegetable per day. One in nine Americans not uncommonly consumes no fruits or vegetables at all. Only 1 in 11 Americans even meets the guidelines for eating the minimum of at least 3 servings per day of vegetables and 2 servings per day of fruit.

Additional information on potential phytonutrient health benefits is available at:

- "Phytochemicals in Produce"

  http://www.ext.colostate.edu/pubs/columnn/nn98026.html

- "Phytochemicals: Vitamins of the Future"

  http://www.ohioline.osu.edu/hyg-fact/5000/5050.html

3.4 Increasing Phytonutrient Intake

Basic strategies for increasing dietary intake of fruits, vegetables, and whole grains include such things as:

- adding chopped fresh fruit to cereal and yogurt

- fortifying soups with beans, fresh greens, carrots, celery, parsley and tomatoes

- keeping fruit available, in sight and in mind for eating

- reaching for freshly squeezed fruit juices instead of coffee or soda

- storing dried fruit (apricots, dates, raisins, prunes, etc) in convenient places for a quick snack at home or work

- using whole grain breads or cereals, etc.

3.5 Major Classes of Phytonutrients

Phytonutrients are classified in a number of different ways, however there is no single, commonly accepted method for doing so. Major classes of phytonutrients are:

- carotenoids

- phenolic acids

- flavonoids (polyphenols)

- phytosterols

- phytoestrogens/isoflavones

- sulfur containing compounds
  - indols
  - isothiocyanates
  - sulforaphane/glucosinolates
  - thiosulfonates

- terpenes

The phytonutrient/phytochemical content of selected foods is available from the USDA Nutrient Data Laboratory at:
http://www.nal.usda.gov/fnic/foodcomp

Phytonutrients in each of the above class are discussed in sections 3.5.1-3.5.5.

3.5.1 Carotenoids

Today, the most information on phytonutrients appears to be available for carotenoids. Over 600 carotenoids occur naturally in various food sources, chiefly in the orange, red, and yellow pigmented fruits and vegetables. Fruits and vegetables that are high in carotenoids are regarded as potentially protective against cancers, cardiovascular diseases, cataracts and age related macular degeneration.

Some of the major carotenoids of interest and their food sources include:

- alpha carotene (carrots)

- astaxanthin (red pigment concentrated in marine animals and fish such as salmon, trout, crab and shrimp)

- beta carotene (broccoli, cantelope, leafy green and yellow vegetables, pumpkin, and sweet potatoes)

- cryptoxanthin (apricots, citrus fruits, and peaches)

- lutein (leafy green vegetables such as collards, kale, spinach and turnip greens)

- lycopene (tomato products, pink or red grapefruit and watermelon)

- zeaxanthin (citrus fruits, eggs, and green vegetables)

Some of the evidence that carotenoids are disease preventive includes the following:

- each increment above 3 daily servings of fruits and vegetables may be equated with a 22% decrease in the risk of stroke

- elderly men with the highest intake of dark green and yellow vegetables are reported to have around a 40-50% decrease in the risk of heart disease and a 70% lower risk of cancer

- men with the highest consumption of tomato products are reported to have around 30-40% decrease in the risk of prostate cancer

- individuals with the highest intake of spinach or collard greens (high in lutein) are reported to have a 40-50% decrease in age related macular degeneration, the leading cause of blindness in the elderly.

Both alpha and beta carotene possess vitamin A activity and are converted in the body into vitamin A. Beta carotene is regarded as the most active of the two in terms of anti-oxidant activity with alpha carotene being around 50% less active.

Women with the highest intakes of fruits and vegetables rich in beta carotene are reported to have a 22% reduction in the risk of a heart attack and a 40% reduction in the risk of stroke.

Lycopene, lutein, and zeaxanthin do not convert to vitamin A but are reported (especially lycopene and lutein) to be active against breast, colorectal, lung, prostate, and uterine cancers. Consumption of tomato based products containing lycopene, for example, is associated with a decreased risk of several cancers, but the evidence appears to be strongest for cancers of the prostate, lung and stomach.

Lycopene consumption via foods also has been reported to be associated with a significant decrease in cardiovascular disease. This decrease is believed to be the result, at least in part, of a reduction of serum low density lipoprotein cholesterol and total cholesterol produced by lycopene as well as its antioxidant activity.

Foods considered to be rich in lycopene content include:

Food	Lycopene content[*]
• ½ cup tomato sauce	22
• ¾ cup tomato juice	20
• 2 tablespoons tomato paste	18
• ¾ cup vegetable juice cocktail	18
• ¼ cup tomato puree	10

- ½ cup chopped raw tomato   8

- 1 cup watermelon chunks   7

- 2 tablespoons ketchup   5

- 1 guava   5

- ½ pink grapefruit   4

* in milligrams

Astaxanthin is regarded as a very potent antioxidant having some ten times the activity as that of other carotenoids, and being one hundred times more effective in trapping damaging free radicals compared with vitamin E. It also is reported to be the most effective carotenoid in terms of reducing mammary tumors in mice. Astaxanthin appears to be one of the most effective anti-inflammatory and antiaging carotenoids studied to date in animals.

It has been recognized for some time that individuals who consume dark green vegetables such as spinach, kale, and collared greens have increased levels of lutein and zeaxanthin in their blood associated have a lowered incidence of cataracts and age related macular degeneration and blindness, especially the elderly. Eating at least three servings of foods rich in lutein and zeaxanthin is reported to reduce the incidence of cataracts in seven out of eight elderly Americans. While darker greens are a good source of lutein, they contain much less zeaxanthin which is considered to be the more important of the two in preventing such eye disease. However, lutein is converted in the body into zeaxanthin and both substances are concentrated in the macula of the eye, the center area involved in visual acuity. Yellow, yellow/green, and orange foods are regarded as among the richest sources of both these carotenoids.

The xanthophylls (cryptoxanthin, zeaxanthin, etc.) appear to be somewhat more tissue/organ specific in terms of disease protective activity. Cryptoxanthin, for example, is regarded as more protective against vaginal, uterine and cervical cancers. On the other hand, zeaxanthin appears to be more active against age related macular degeneration. Also, the xanthophylls are reported to protect vitamins A and E and other carotenoids against oxidation and degradation.

Carotenoids from food are not easily assimilated into the body after ingestion because they are tightly bound in the foods in which they are contained. Therefore, it is best to cook, puree, or juice such foods in order to release their carotenoid content to aid absorption. Also, because carotenoids are fat soluble, consuming them with fats/oils increases their uptake/assimilation from the intestine.

3.5.2 Phenolic acids

Phenolic acids are among the most abundant antioxidants in nature. They are found in most fruits, vegetables, and herbs. In fact, the preservative properties of herbs are considered to be chiefly due to their inherent phenolic acid content. Phenolic acids also are found in berries as well as whole grains.

They are regarded not only as potent antioxidants but also somewhat specialized in terms of activity. For example, some are reported to prevent oxidation of low density lipoprotein cholesterol, and thus may be useful in helping prevent cardiovascular diseases. Others are regarded as cancer preventive owing to their ability to:

- block the formation of nitrosamines (cancer producing compounds) from dietary nitrates and nitrates found in meats

- removing free radical producing minerals such as copper and iron, and increasing cancer cell death (apoptosis)

Chief phenolic acids of currrent interest include anthocyanins, caffeic acid, catechins, cinnamic, chlorogenic, coumaric, ellagic, ferrulic, malic, piperic, piponylic, quercetin, salicylic, tannic, and vanillin.

Fruits that are colored blue, purple, or red are considered to be rich sources of caffeic, chlorogenic, and coumaric acids. Ellagic acid found in red fruits has been reported to be effective against chemically induced cancers of the esophagus, liver, lung, and skin in animal models. Apples are an important source of caffeic, coumaric, ellagic, and malic acids. The skin of red apples contains an important flavonoid, quercetin, which is related to the phenolic acids. Apple extracts also are reported to inhibit cancer tumor growth in animals, and improve lung function in men.

3.5.3 Flavonoids/Polyphenols

Flavonoids constitute a large family of polyphenol phytonutrients that include catechins in tea, quercetin in apples/onions/teas/wine, and anthocyanins in red fruits and vegetables. Over 4,000 flavonoids have now been identified in various fruits, vegetables, nuts, seeds, tea and wine.

Major disease preventative activities of the flavonoids include:

* lowering the infection rate

* improving immune function

* preventing cardiovascular diseases and cancers

* protecting against allergies

* reducing oxidative stress and cellular free radical damage

Evidence that flavonoids are cardioprotective, for example, includes the following:

* overall flavonoid consumption is linked to a lower risk of heart disease, and men with the highest flavonoid intake have a 58% lower risk of heart disease

* individuals with the highest flavonoid intake also have a lower mortality from heart disease, 27% lower for women and 33% for men

* flavonoids block the angiotensin converting enzyme that controls blood pressure

* flavonoids reduce platelet stickiness and aggregation via inhibition of the cyclooxygnease enzyme system

* flavonoids appear to protect the vascular system, strengthening the capillaries, and promoting vasodilation, aiding circulation

Anthocyanins, anthocyaninidins, and proanthocyaninidins are polyphenolic phytonutrients found in red fruits along with ellagic and other phenolic acids. Red berries, especially their skins, are considered to be excellent sources of antioxidants that are protective against free radical cell damage, and chronic disease.

Catechins also are regarded as important polyphenolic phytonutrients found in tea. They are considered to be highly active antioxidants and disease preventative compounds. Available research indicates that tea catechins and other phytonutrients may be helpful in:

- ameliorating allergies

- enhancing immune function

- increasing the body's metabolic rate, fat burning, and weight loss

- inhibiting infections

- lowering blood pressure and the risk of stroke

- maintaining bone density/decreasing fracture rate

- preventing cancer.

Drinking green tea may protect against cancers of the lymph and prostate glands by inducing programmed cell death or apoptosis of cancer cells. Catechins also may protect against prostate cancer by blocking androgen hormone receptors in prostate tissue. Catechins appear to have similar activity against hormone dependent breast cancer.

Red grapes and red wines also are reported to contain significant amounts of flavonoids, particularly proanthocyanindins, resveratrol, and ellagic acid. Resveratrol is concentrated chiefly in the skin of red grapes, and chlorogenic and other phenolic acids are found chiefly in grape flesh. These phenolic acids and flavonoids are reported to contribute to red wine's ability to help prevent cardiovascular disease and stroke. Other beverages with a significant content of phenolic acids and flavonoids, such as beer and grape juice also are reported to help prevent heart disease.

Resveratrol research indicates that this phytonutrient also may inhibit tumor growth, prevent cancer of the breast, colon, and liver, and may also decrease heart disease due to its anti-inflammatory properties. It also may exert some of its disease prevention through action as a phytoestrogen.

3.5.4 Sulfur Containing Compounds

Cruciferous (meaning bearing a flowery cross) green vegetables such as broccoli, cabbage, cauliflower, and brussels sprouts are regarded as among the more important food groups for disease prevention. These vegetables belong to the family Brassicaceae. Brassicae, a related group of vegetables, includes asparagus, garlic, onions, and scallions. Each of these vegetables is considered to provide a unique sulfur containing phytonutrients possessing disease preventative activity.

Sulfur chemical bonds contained in these phytonutrients are regarded as important because they may help transform harmful chemicals into substances that can be more easily eliminated from the body (a process called detoxification).

Consumption of cruciferous vegetables is associated with a reduced incidence of hormone dependent cancers as well as cancer of the bladder.

3.5.4.1 Indoles

Indole-3-carbinol (13C) is considered to be another important cancer preventative compound found in broccoli, brussel sprouts, cabbage and kale. It is reported to inhibit estrogen dependent breast cancer.

3.5.4.2 Sulforaphane/Glucosinolates

Glucosinolates are found in foods throughout the broccoli and mustard families with the highest concentrations reported in cabbage, cauliflower, broccoli, and brussels sprouts. Calcium D-glucarate produced from the glucosinolate, sulforaphane, is considered to be an important inhibitor of breast cancer, and may also increase the effectiveness of standard chemotherapy for breast cancer.

3.5.4.3 Isothiocyanates

Isothiocynates are biotransformation products produced from sulforaphane. These phytonutrients are found principally in cabbage, kale, mustard seeds and greens, and may be helpful in preventing lung and esophageal cancers in smokers. Isothiocyanates may be effective against cancers of the gastrointestinal tract, including the colon, mouth, pharynx, stomach and rectum.

3.5.4.4 Thiosulfonates

Garlic, onions, chives, leaks, scallions, and shallots are members of the Attiaceae family of vegetables. Garlic and onions produce phytonutrients called thiosulfonates (allylic sulfides, ajoenes, mercaptocysteines, etc). Garlic and onion have been used over the years for reducing blood fats, lowering blood pressure, inhibiting platelet clumping/blood clotting, promoting vascular relaxation through release of nitric oxide, and preventing cardiovascular disease. Individuals who consume garlic routinely in their food also are reported to have a lower incidence of stomach cancer, presumably due to inhibition of the microbe, Helicobacter pylori, regarded as a primary causative agent in stomach cancer.

A host of new studies provide reasonably good evidence that garlic and its organic allyl sulfur components are effective inhibitors of the cancer process. Of the 37 observational studies reviewed by the NCI, 28 showed cancer protective effects. The evidence is regarded as particularly strong for a link between garlic and the prevention of prostate and stomach cancers.

Peeling garlic releases an enzyme called allinase that starts a series of chemical reactions that produce diallyl disulfides (DADs). These compounds also are formed when raw garlic is cut or crushed. However, if garlic is cooked immediately after peeling, cutting or crushing, the allinase is inactivated and the cancer fighting benefit is lost. Therefore, one should wait around 5-10 minutes between peeling and cooking garlic to allow the allinase reaction to occur. Processing garlic into powder or garlic oil also releases cancer fighting substances.

Some of the garlic compounds currently under investigation as anticancer substances include: allin (responsible for garlic odor), alline (odorless), ajoene (naturally occurring disulfide), diallyl disulfides (DADS), diallyl trisulfide (DAT), S-allylcysteine (SAC), organosulfur compounds, and allyl sulfur compounds.

A NCI fact sheet: "Garlic and Cancer Prevention" is available at: http://cancer.gov/newscenter/pressreleases/garlic

A report on "Garlic: Effects on Cardiovascular Risks and Disease, Protective Effects Against Cancer, and Clinical Adverse Effects" is available at: http://ahrq.gov/clinic/tp/garlictp.htm

3.5.4.5 Terpenes

This class includes key phytonutrients such as perillyl alcohol (found in cherries) and limonene (found in citrus fruits) which have been demonstrated to have significant anticancer activity in animals.

3.5.5 Phytosterols

Most green and yellow vegetables, whole grains, nuts, seeds, soy, fresh and dried peas, and saw palmetto berries are reported to be good sources for plant sterols (phytosterols). These plant sterols compete with dietary cholesterol and block its absorption. A review of clinical trails to date indicates that phytosterols lower total blood cholesterol by an average of 10%. As a result, phytosterols have been added to soft margarine products to make them functional foods with FDA approved health claims for lowering cholesterol.

Six major phytosterols, (each in varying amounts of avenasterol, campesterol, stigmasterol, oryzanol, beta sitosterol, and gamma sitosterol) are found in various food sources. Beta sitosterol, stigmasterol, and campesterol are the most commonly found ones in whole grains.

Brown rice and other whole grains are reported to contain a greater variety of phytosterols compared with most other foods and are recommended for this reason as an important part of any dietary plan.

Phytosterols also are reported to block the development of tumors of the breast, colon, and prostate glands in animals and thus may play a role in the prevention of these cancers in humans.

3.5.6 Phytoestrogens/Isoflavones

Phytoestrogens are a group of isoflavones and lignans that appear to protect against cancer, cardiovascular disease and osteoporosis. For additional information, see:
http://www.som.tulane.edu/eeme/eehome/basics/phytoestrogens

Isoflavones, a phenol subclass of phytonutrients, are found in soybeans and other legumes. They are chemically related to the flavonoids. The most widely known isoflavones are genistein and daidzen which can be found in soy beans and their products. They are reported to help prevent cardiovascular disease and cancer and to protect against spinal bone loss.

Available evidence now indicates that these natural phytoestrogens found in soybeans and many other plant foods may significantly reduce hot flashes and vaginal dryness as well as increase bone density after menopause. Soy isoflavones also act as weak estrogens, in the body, substituting for natural estrogen, and blocking surplus estrogen that may be responsible for hormonal imbalances and cancer. Isoflavones also appear to reduce prostate tumor growth and breast cancer in animals suggesting cancer protective potential as well. For additional information, see: http://www.ars.usda.gov/is/pr/2001/010928.htm

Soy isoflavones are considered to be important phytonutrients that aid in lowering total blood cholesterol and low density lipoprotein cholesterol (LDL-C), while raising high density lipoprotein cholesterol (HDL-C). In addition, isoflavones are regarded as excellent free radical scavengers. Thus, soy isoflavones appear to play a significant role in reducing the risk of cardiovascular disease in populations that consume higher levels of soy products in their diets.

Foods high in isoflavones include:

Food (serving)	Isoflavones in milligrams
• textured soy protein granules (1/4 Cup)	60
• roasted soy nuts (1/4 cup)	60
• tempeh (1/2 cup)	35
• tofu, low fat and regular (1/2 cup)	35
• regular soy milk (1/2 cup)	30
• roasted soy butter (1 serving)	17
• meatless soy burger crumbles (1 serving)	9

Phytic acid, another soy component, binds calcium and iron in the intestines impairing their absorption. While regarded as an antinutrient in this regard, iron binding may be considered one of the ways soy may protect against breast, colon, prostate, and perhaps other cancers as well since cancer cells rely on iron for their growth and growth is slowed when not enough iron is available. In addition, too much iron can promote cardiovascular disease with iron acting as a free radical, damaging vascular tissue and oxidizing LDL-C which produces adverse circulatory effects.

3.6 Whole Grain Phytonutrients

Whole grains refers to grains that are minimally processed and retain their content of important antioxidants, phytates, phytosterols, and phytoestrogens. In addition to such phytonutrients, whole grains are an important source of essential fatty acids, fiber, complex carbohydrates, essential B vitamins, vitamin E, and trace antioxidant minerals such as copper, manganese, selenium and zinc.

Whole grains include barley, bulgar, millet, oats, rye, wheat, etc. They are always cooked or processed before being eaten.

Whole grains consist of three basic layers. First there is the bran, or outer coating/layer that consists of mostly indigestible complex carbohydrates. Vitamins and minerals are located just under the bran layer, and most of the water soluble ones are lost from the grain when it is processed and the bran is removed.

Then there is the second, germ layer, which contains oils and fat soluble vitamins such as vitamin E and the tocotrienols, classified as members of the E family of vitamins.

Lastly, there is the endosperm layer which is regarded as the "sweetest" part of the grain because it consists chiefly of stored, digestible starch and enzymes that break down starch into sugars.

Whole grains are protected by the bran layer during growth and until environmental conditions turn favorable for sprouting. The new plant is sprouted from the germ layer. Vitamins and minerals, starch, etc from the endosperm layer support the sprouting process and initial growth of the grain seed until the chlorophyll rich stalk and leaves form and take over food production and supply for the new plant.

Barley is best known as a soup ingredient. It is a rich source of tocotrienols, powerful antioxidants that help prevent cardiovasculart disease and cancer. It also contains beta glucon, a soluble fiber that helps reduce blood lipid levels. One cup of barley is reported to contain around 6 grams of fiber.

Bulgar is wheat kernels that have been steamed, dried, and crushed. This whole grain contains ferulic acid, lignans, and other antioxidant compounds that help protect against cancer. Its carbohydrates have a low glycemic index that helps control blood sugar levels in diabetics. Also, it is high in fiber, containing around twice as much as an equal portion of oatmeal.

Brown rice also is abundant in fiber, complex carbohydrates and B vitamins. It is reported to have 10 times more fiber than white rice, and its bran contains oryzanol, a sterol that helps reduce blood lipid levels.

Other whole grains, also are rich in fiber compared to their refined counterparts, and they contain a host of other nutrients and phytonutrients. For example, one cup of oatmeal is reported to deliver 4 grams of dietary fiber with twice the cholesterol lowering power as the highest wheat bran cereal plus 56 milligrams of magnesium.

Whole grains are considered to be protective against a number of disorders such as cardiovascular disease, diabetes mellitus and stroke. Individuals who eat the least whole grain foods/fiber are reported to have the greatest risk for a heart attack as well as a fatal outcome from such an attack. Men who are in the top 20% of fiber intake in their diet are reported to have 1/3 less chance of dying from a heart attack. Dark bread, whole grain breakfast cereals, cooked oatmeal, wheat germ, brown rice, bran, bulgar, coucous, and kaska appear to offer the best whole grain protection in this regard. In addition, eating whole grains is reported to be associated with reduced risk of type 2 diabetes mellitus in the elderly. Studies also indicate that women eating the most whole grain foods, garlic and onions enjoy a significant reduction in breast cancer.

Whole grains are low in fat, contain no cholesterol, are high in dietary fiber and vitamins, and are a good source of minerals. While whole grains contain significant amounts of starch, they also contain 10-15% protein, and are a good source of health promoting phytonutrients.

Individuals who consume whole grains are reported to live a much healthier and longer life. Those that consume at least one serving of whole grain foods a day, primarily as bread and breakfast cereal, are reported to have a significantly lower rate of death from all causes. Whole grain bread and cereal intake is reported to be directly linked to a decreased risk of coronary heart disease, a leading cause of death for both men and women in the United States. Although soluble fiber in whole grains is believed to play a significant role, antioxidants, phytic acid, lectins, phenolic compounds, amylase inhibitors, saponins, lignans, and other factors in whole grains may play a role as well.

Whole grains also are rich sources of a number of phytonutrients that are reported to block DNA damage from free radicals and suppress cancer cell growth. The dietary fiber in whole grains increases fecal bulk and speeds food transit in the intestines decreasing the opportunity for mutagens to damage cells and cause cancer of the digestive tract. Lignan phytoestrogens in whole grains also may protect against hormonally mediated diseases such as cancers of the breast and prostate. In addition, individuals who consume the most whole grain cereal fiber are reported to have about a 35% lower risk of developing non-insulin-dependent type 2 diabetes mellitus. Lignans in whole grains also may protect against hormonally mediated cancers of the breast and prostate.

Additional information is available at:

http://www.nlm.nih.gov/medlineplus/news/fullstory_11953.html

Research indicates that individuals who eat the most whole grains tend to weigh less, and are healthier, live longer and have a lower death rate from all causes. In addition, whole grain intake is directly related to a decreased risk of cardiovascular disease and stroke. This may be due to soluble fiber in whole grains that lower blood cholesterol, as well as phytonutrient content.

Whole grains also offer significant antioxidant protection against free radical damage particularly oats, rye and wheat. The whole grain antioxidants, caffeic and ferulic acids appear to be potent anticancer phytonutrients. Wheat varieties most effective in killing cancer cells are reported to have 10 times as much caffeic and ferulic acids as the least effective types. And mice fed wheat rich in caffeic and ferulic acids are reported to be 60% less likely to develop cancer of the colon.

The US Surgeon General's goal for all Americans is to consume at least 3 servings a day of whole grains but the nation's average is now only about half a serving a day. Only 13% of Americans include at least one serving of whole grains in their daily diets. Most individuals should start the day with a whole grain, high fiber content cereal and/or bread for breakfast. Consideration also should be given to consuming whole grain foods at other meals.

The FDA now allows food manufacturers to claim health benefits for products that contain at least 51% whole grain by weight and less than 3% of fat per serving. This claim is as follows:

"Diets rich in whole grain foods and other plant foods low in total fat, saturated fat and cholesterol may help reduce the risk of heart disease and certain cancers".

3.7 Flaxseed Phytonutrients

A diet rich in flaxseed is reported to decrease size, aggressiveness and severity of prostate tumors in mice. Also, in men with prostate cancer, flaxseed added to their diet may decrease testosterone as well as PSA (prostate specific antigen) levels in blood. This is believed to be due to flaxseed's phytonutrient content.

3.8 Phytonutrients/Cancer Prevention

Research indicates that phytonutrients in fruits, vegetables, seeds and nuts may affect various metabolic pathways important in cancer prevention in a number of ways, namely:

- coumarins, flavonoids, and triterpenoids may block a carcinogen's initiation of the cancer producing process

- sulfides and isoflavones may block further tumor promotion once cancer formation has been initiated

- carotenoids, flavonoids, phenolic acids, terpenes, and tocopherols, acting as antioxidants, may block oxidative free radical damage and tumor promotion

- flavonoids, phenolic acids, salicylates, and sulfur containing compounds may block the action of prostaglandins on tumor promotion

- fiber, lignans, phenolic compounds, phytosterols, isoflavones, and cruciferous indoles may block the effect of steroid hormones on tumor promotion.

While research to date in these regards appears promising, much additional work still is needed to clarify the role of various phytonutrients in the prevention of cancer.

Use the Search sites in the Web resources below for additional information regarding phytonutrients/phytochemicals, namely:

- The Phytonutrient Laboratory

  http://www.barc.usda.gov/bhnrc/pl/index.html

- Food and Nutrition Information Center

  http://www.nal.usda.gov/fnic

- Medlineplus

  http://www.nlm.nih.gov/medlineplus

A "NCI Fact Sheet: Antioxidants and Cancer Prevention" is available at:
http://www.cancer.gov/newscenter/pressreleases/antioxidants

4. Five to Nine a Day: Fruits/ Vegetables/Seeds/Nuts

4.1 Introduction

The National Center for Chronic Disease Prevention and Health Promotion (NCCDPHP) now encourages 5 to 9 servings a day of a variety of fruits and vegetables as the best nutritional way to a healthier lifestyle and a longer life. Individuals are encouraged to try at least one new fruit or vegetable each week to obtain a variety of health benefits. Seeds and nuts also are encouraged to be made part of the diet for their health promoting benefits.

The Surgeon General's Report on Nutrition and Health 1988, noted that 2/3 of all deaths are due to diseases associated with diet. The report also states that the three most important personal habits that influence health are smoking, alcohol consumption and diet. For two out of three adults who do not drink alcohol excessively or smoke, the single most important choice influencing long term health is diet.

In 1997, the World Cancer Research Fund and the American Institute for Cancer Research report, "Food, Nutrition and the Prevention of Cancer: A Global Perspective" stated that recommended diets in conjunction with physical activity and normal "body mass index" could reduce cancer incidence by up to 40%.

The 1989 National Academy of Science report, "Diet and Health: Implications for Reducing Chronic Disease Risk'", projected that 20% of deaths could be avoided by reducing fats, and increasing fruits, vegetables, whole grain

breads and cereals, and legumes (dry beans and peas). For additional information, see:
http://www.cdc.gov/nccdphp/dnpa/5aday/faq/our_health_4.htm

The "Five to Nine a Day for Better Health Program" is a large scale public/private partnership between the fruit and vegetable industry and the US Government. This national nutrition program seeks to increase the number of daily servings Americans eat of fruits and vegetables from five to nine a day. The program is designed to inform Americans that eating fruits and vegetables can improve their health and reduce the risk of cancer, cardiovascular disorders, and other chronic illnesses.

This campaign promotes eating a wide variety of fruits and vegetables every day to help prevent chronic disease and maintain health. Seeds and nuts should be included as well.

4.2 Research Backs Benefits

Numerous research studies and reviews indicate that diets rich in fruits and vegetables are associated with reduced risks for chronic diseases including a number of types of cancer. While more research is needed to clarify issues, the bulk of research available provides sufficient evidence to support these health benefits. One needs to bear in mind however, that research results highlighted in the media often tend to over emphasize the unusual or conflicting results rather than confirming the more prevalent position and more consistent data.

Health benefits are discussed in a report from the Harvard School of Public Health entitled, "Fruits and Vegetables", available at:
http://www.hsph.harvard.edu/nutritionsource/fruits.html

The National Center for Chronic Disease Prevention and Health Promotion report on: "Frequently Asked Questions: The Importance of Fruits and Vegetables" is available at:
http://www.dcd.gov/nccdphp/dnpa/5aday/faq

4.3 Color Your Way/5 to 9 a Day

4.3.1 Introduction

The power of colorful fruits and vegetables to promote good health is now widely recognized. Such is believed largely due to specific phytonutrients found in different colored fruits and vegetables. To obtain the full potential benefits of these phytonutrients, it is advisable to eat a wide variety of different colored fruits and vegetables. When it comes to your health, you likely will fare best with multivaried, multicolored fruits and vegetables on the order of 5 to 9 servings a day.

A summary of fruits and vegetables included in each color group, phytonutrient content, and potential health benefits are available at:
http://www.5aday.org/html/colorway/colorway_home.php
http://www.nal.usda.gov/fnic/etext/000059.html

A diet rich in fruits and vegetables does not require spending a great deal of money. In fact, eating fruits and vegetables not only can be a delicious but also an affordable way to stay healthy according to a report: "5 a Day the Affordable Way" available at:
http://www.cdc.gov/nccdphp/dnpa/5aday/campaign/affordable.htm

A fact sheet on the phytochemical content of fruits and vegetables is available at:
http://ohioline.osu.edu/hyg-fact/5000/5050.html

4.3.2 Blues/Purples

Blue and purple fruits and vegetables contain varying amounts of important health promoting phytonutrients such as anthocyanins and phenolic compounds. These are being researched for their antioxidant and anticancer activities, and their ability to reduce cardiovascular disease and slow down the aging process. Blue and purple fruits and vegetables are recommended in "5 to 9 a day" dietary regimens.

Key blue and purple food sources for anthocyanin and phenolic compounds are:

Anthocyanins

Phenolic compounds

- Blackberries
- Black currants
- Blueberries
- Elderberries
- Purple grapes
- Purple figs
- Purple peppers

- Dried plums (prunes)
- Eggplant
- Plums
- Raisins

Additional information and recipes for some of these blue and purple food sources are available at:
http://www.cdc.gov/nccdphp/dnpa/5aday/campaign/color/blues/htm

4.3.3 Greens

Green fruits and vegetables contain phytonutrients considered important for lowering cancer risk, improving vision, and maintaining strong bones and teeth. They also are recommended in "5 to 9 a day" dietary regimens.

Green leafy vegetables such as spinach, romaine lettuce, collared greens, kale, and broccoli are good sources for the carotenoids, lutein and zeaxanthin, which are powerful antioxidants. Lutein and zeaxanthin are being studied for their role in helping maintain good vision and preventing cataracts and age related macular degeneration.

Indoles are another group of phytonutrients found in cruciferous vegetables such as broccoli, cauliflower, cabbage, and brussels sprouts. Indoles are being evaluated for their potential role in helping protect against breast cancer (which affects one out of every eight women) and prostate cancer (which affects one out of every six men) in the United States. In a recent study, men who consumed cruciferous vegetables at least three times a week had a 40-50% reduction in the risk for prostate cancer.

Key green food sources for these phytonutrients are as follows:

<u>Lutein/zeaxanthin</u>

- Broccoli
- Collard greens
- Green peas
- Honeydew melon
- Kale

- Kiwi
- Mustard greens
- Romaine lettuce
- Turnip greens
- Spinach

<u>Indoles</u>

- Arugula
- Bok choy
- Broccoli
- Brussels sprouts
- Cabbage

- Cauliflower
- Kale
- Swiss chard
- Turnips

Additional information and recipes for some of these green food sources are available at:
http://www.cdc.gov/nccdphp/dnpa/5aday/campaign/color/greens.htm

4.3.4 Oranges/Yellows

Orange and bright yellow fruits and vegetables contain the carotenoid, beta carotene and as well as flavonoids. They are recommended in a "5 to 9 a day" dietary regimen. Sweet potatoes, carrots, and pumpkins all contain beta carotene. Citrus fruits, such as oranges, grapefruits, and tangerines contain flavonoids plus vitamin C.

Beta carotene is a potent antioxidant being researched along with vitamin C and E for its role in reducing the risk of cancer, cardiovascular disease, cataracts, and age related macular degeneration, as well as its ability to boost the immune system and slow aging.

Sunlight breaks down carotenoids such as beta carotene rather easily, when vegetables are cut up. Lightly cooking food makes carotenoids easier to absorb from the intestines.

Flavonoids seem to work as a team with vitamin C. They are being evaluated for their potential role in reducing the risk of cancer and cardiovascular disease as well as in strengthening bones and teeth, helping heal wounds and keeping skin healthy.

Key food sources for beta carotene and flavonoids are as follows:

Beta-carotene	Flavonoids
	• Apricots
Fruits	• Grapefruits
	• Lemons
• Apricots	• Nectarines
• Cantaloupe	• Oranges
• Mangos	• Papaya
• Peaches	• Peaches

Vegetables

- Butternut squash
- Carrots
- Pumpkin
- Sweet potato

- Pears (yellow)
- Pineapple
- Pepper (yellow)
- Raisins (yellow)

Additional information and recipes for some of these orange and yellow food sources are available at:
http://www.cdc.gov/nccdphp/dnpa/5aday/campaign/color/orange_yellow.htm

4.3.5 Reds/Pinks

Red colored fruits and vegetables are rich sources of the key carotenoid, lycopene and the flavonoid anthocyanin, both potent antioxidants important in the prevention of cardiovascular disease and cancer.

Lycopene gives rise to the red color in tomatoes. Cooked tomatoes (sauce or paste) result in better absorption of lycopene and greater health benefits. A small amount of fat also increases the absorption of lycopene. Lycopene is being evaluated for its role in helping to reduce the risk of several types of cancer, including prostate cancer (the second leading cause of cancer death in American men, killing over 30,000 annually).

Anthocyanins are being evaluated for their ability to prevent cardiovascular disease and cancer, as well as their anti-inflammatory activity and ability to delay or prevent several diseases associated with the aging process.

Additional information and recipes for selected red and pink foods are available at:
http://www.cdc.gov/nccdphp/dnpa/5aday/campaign/color/reds.htm

Key food sources for lycopene and anthocyanins are:

<u>Lycopene</u>

- Grapefruit (pink)
- Guava
- Papaya

- Tomato/tomato products
- Watermelon

<u>Anthocyanins</u>

<u>Fruits</u>

- Apples (red)
- Cherries (sweet)
- Cranberries
- Raspberries (red)
- Strawberries

<u>Vegetables</u>

- Beets
- Beans (kidney)
- Cabbage (red)
- Onions (red)
- Peppers (red)

4.3.6 Whites/Browns/Tans

White, brown and tan fruits and vegetables contain varying amounts of health promoting sulfur compounds (e.g. allicin, sulforaphane, etc.). One of the more interesting in this group is allicin. Research is being conducted to show how allicin in garlic and onions may help lower blood cholesterol and blood pressure as well as increase the body's ability to fight infections. Other sulfur containing compounds of the sulforaphane group are being investigated for their anticancer properties.

Good food sources for sulfur containing phytonutrients in this class are:

Fruits   Vegetables

- Bananas   - Cauliflower

- Brown pears   - Chives

- Dates   - Garlic

- Nectarines (white)   - Leeks

- Peaches (white)   - Onions

                                          - Scallions

                                          - Shallots

                                          - Potatoes (white)

                                          - Turnips

Garlic, onions and leeks may be lacking in colorful hues, however, they remain important sources of key phytonutrients. The National 5 to 9 a Day for Better Health Partnership recommends flavoring salads, sandwiches, and main dishes with garlic, onions, scallions and/or leeks to be consumed each day.

Additional information and recipes for white, brown and tan foods are available at:
http://www.cdc.gov/nccdphp.dnpa/5aday/campaign/color/white.htm

4.4 Fruits/Vegetables

Because of their large numbers, all fruits/vegetables available today cannot be discussed. As a result, only a select group of 36 commonly consumed fruits and vegetables are reviewed. Information on others may be obtained by searching Web resources provided in Chapter 7. The 36 fruits/vegetables are reviewed alphabetically in sections 4.4.1-4.4.36 respectively.

The nutrient content given for each fruit or vegetable reviewed, while regarded as generally representative, may vary significantly from variety to variety, season and soil conditions, as well as a host of other factors, and therefore should be regarded accordingly.

4.4.1 Apples

The average American is reported to eat around 120 apples each year. Serving size is 1 medium apple (154 grams/5.5 ounces). Each apple is reported to contain around 80 calories, 20 grams of carbohydrate, 5 grams of dietary fiber (20% DV) and 8% DV vitamin C.

Apples should be kept available as a low calorie snack, and one should consider including them in a lunch, on a break or as an addition to your salad. Try baking an apple with a touch of cinnamon for desert, or adding chopped apples to your whole grain cereal for breakfast. Use applesauce instead of shortening in your baked goods to reduce fats and calories.

Apples convey significant health benefits that appear to bear out the old saying "an apple a day keeps the doctor away". Research indicates that:

- the phytonutrient, quercetin, found principally in apple skins, may provide a method for preventing or treating prostate cancer, and reducing the risk of lung cancer.

- quercetin also decreases pancreatic tumor growth, and increases cancer cell destruction (apoptosis), in animals

- phytonutrients in apples inhibit the growth of colon and liver cancer cells in vitro. One hundred grams of unpeeled fresh apple, about 2/3 of a medium sized apple, provides the antioxidant activity of 1,500 milligrams of vitamin C

- lung cancer was found to be 46% lower among those whose diets contained the highest amounts of apple flavonoids

- individuals who ate at least 2 apples per week had a 22-32% lower risk of developing asthma, and apple eaters are reported to have better lung function

- daily consumption of apples and apple juice may help slow the oxidation and free radical production process that is involved in plaque build up that leads to heart disease. In addition, high consumption of flavonoids from apples is reported to be directly related to the lowest risk for coronary heart disease mortality

- individuals who ate the most apples had the lowest risk of thrombotic stroke, attributed to the broad phytonutrient content (quercetin, catechins, etc.) in apples.

Information on apples, selection, storage, preparation, varieties, use in a "5 to 9 a day" plan, and recipes are available at:
http://www.cdc.gov/nccdphp/dnpa/5aday/month/apple.htm

Additional information regarding apple health benefits is available at:
http://www.usapple.org/educators/research/research.shtml

4.4.2 Asparagus

Asparagus is sometimes referred to as the aristocrat of vegetables. It can be found in green and white varieties, more common in the US and Europe, respectively. White asparagus is grown under the soil, and is shielded from the sun's rays. Therefore, it does not produce the chlorophyll necessary to produce a green color.

Serving size is 3.5 ounces raw asparagus (8 spears). A serving has only around 22 calories and is rich in potassium (around 302 milligrams). It provides 55% DV of vitamin C, 34% DV of folate, 20% DV vitamin E, 18% DV of vitamin A, around 8-10% DV of fiber, and 3 grams of protein, 4 grams of carbohydrate, and no fat. Asparagus is a well balanced nutritious vegetable.

Asparagus should be included in any "5 to 9 a day" plan. It can be served cold with a low fat dressing, added to a salad, served as a side dish or as a treat with fresh lemon juice. Steamed asparagus compliments any meal, and leftovers can be used to create a delicious soup.

Additional information on asparagus, storage, preparation, inclusion in a "5 to 9 a day" plan, and recipes are available at:
http://www.cdc.gov/nccdphp/dnpa/5aday/month/asparagus.htm

4.4.3 Bananas

Bananas are inexpensive and the most popular fresh fruit in the United States. They are reported to have high carbohydrate and potassium contents, which makes them a fruit of choice for athletes and individuals who exercise regularly.

Serving size is 1 medium banana (126 grams/4.5 ounces). One serving contains 110 calories, 400 milligrams of potassium (11% DV), 29 grams of carbohydrate (10% DV), 15% DV vitamin C, 4 grams of fiber, and no fat or sodium.

As part of a "5 to 9 a day" plan, bananas may be sliced in cereal, yogurt, or in a salad, and consumed as a no fat snack, or eaten as a desert

Additional information on bananas, selection, storage, varieties, inclusion in a "5 to 9 a day" plan and recipes are available at: http://www.cdc.gov/nccdphp/dnpa/5aday/month/banana.htm

4.4.4 Beets

American beets are descended from a wild slender rooted plant that grew abundantly in ancient Southern Europe. In these ancient civilizations only the green leaves of the beet plant were eaten. In the 1800's beets gained significant popularity as a food in the United States. Modern day beets are a root vegetable with two parts, the root and the edible green leaves. They belong to the botanical species Beta vulgaris, which also includes sugar beets (processed for commercial sugar) and Swiss chard (grown for their greens).

Fresh beets are higher in nutritive value than their canned counterparts. They are low in calories and high in vitamin C, folate, potassium, fiber, and protein. Beet greens also are high in vitamin C (30% RDA in ½ cup cooked greens), and vitamin A (46% RDA in ½ cup cooked greens). One cup of cooked beets contains 75 calories, 0.3 gram total fat (0.1 gram each of saturated, monounsaturated, and polyunsaturated fat), 3.4 grams dietary fiber, 3 grams protein, 17 grams carbohydrate, no cholesterol, 131 milligrams sodium, 136 milligrams folate, and 519 milligrams potassium. Beets are notable for their sweetness and they are reported to have the highest sugar content of any vegetable.

Red beets not only contain the antioxidants, vitamins A and C, but also anthocyanins that help control high blood pressure and protect against cardiovascular disease, diabetes and inflammation.

Beets also contain another phytonutrient, betaine (trimethylglycine), related to choline (tetramethylglycine). Betaine functions very closely with choline, folic acid, vitamin B-12, and a form of the amino acid methionine, known as SAMe (S-adenosylmethionine) as a methyl donor. Donation of methyl groups by betaine is considered to be important for proper liver function, cellular replication, and detoxification reactions as well as in protecting kidneys from damage.

Betaine also may play a role in reducing blood homocysteine levels believed to be involved in cardiovascular disease, atherosclerosis, and osteoporosis. Because of its ability to help the liver process fats (lipids), and protect the liver against chemical damage and fatty infiltration, the first stage of liver damage from excessive consumption of alcohol, betaine is often referred to as the "lipotropic factor". In clinical trials, betaine has been shown to produce significant improvement in alcohol related liver disease in its early stages.

Additional information on beets, selection, health benefits, storage, varieties, inclusion in a "5 to 9 a day" plan and recipes are available at:
http://www.umext.maine.edu/onlinepubs/htmpubs/4252.htm
http://www.healthwell.com/healthnotes/Supp/Betaine.cfm

4.4.5 Berries

4.4.5.1 Introduction

Berries have origins both in Europe and America. Native Americans were among the first to incorporate berries into their diets and lifestyles. Owing to their nutritional value and health promoting properties, berries have become appreciated worldwide. They signify summer as the warmer months are the peak harvest time for these fruits. While many varieties of berries have come into the marketplace in recent years, they are too numerous to discuss individually. Therefore, discussion is limited to five commonly consumed ones, namely: blackberries, blueberries, cranberries, raspberries and strawberries.

All five types are suitable for juice, jam, or preserves, or they may be eaten raw. Each type is regarded as brimming with significant levels of vitamin C, potassium, dietary fiber, and disease preventive phytonutrients. Berries are most suitable for a "5 to 9 a day" plan. Fresh berries can be used in many ways such as toppings for low fat ice cream, pancakes, and waffles. They can be added to cereals for breakfast, or incorporated into fruits salads and compotes, or in muffins and pancakes. Or they may be combined in a frozen fruit kabob. A frozen berry smoothie also can be made for a refreshing treat during the day.

Additional berry information, varieties, storage, freezing, preparing, health benefits, inclusion in a "5 to 9 a day" plan, and recipes are available at:
http://www.cdc.gov/nccdphp/dnpa/5aday/month/berries.htm
http://www.oregon-berries.com
http://www.cranberryinstitute.org/healthresearch.htm
http://www.calstrawberry.com/health/factsheet.asp

4.4.5.2 Blackberries

Archeologists in Denmark, England and Ireland, have provided evidence that blackberries and raspberries were part of the diet of Viking era people. Blackberries are reported to have significant antioxidant activity that may help prevent cardiovascular disease, cancer, and other age related disorders considered to be due, at least in part, to free radical cell damage. Blackberry jam is a favorite of Americans. In recent years consumption of blackberries has soared in popularity and they are served in many homes and fine restaurants. Oregon, Texas, California and Washington provide the bulk of blackberries to the US market.

Serving size is 1 cup (144 grams, 5 ounces). A serving contains 60 calories, 1 gram fat, no saturated fat or cholesterol or sodium, 37 grams total carbohydrate (4% DV), 6 grams dietary fiber (22% DV), 11 grams sugars, 1 gram protein, 50% DV Vitamin C, and 4% DV calcium and iron.

4.4.5.3 Blueberries

The American Indians valued wild blueberries and called them "star berries" because their calyx forms a five pointed star at the blossom of each berry.

Indian legends hold that the "Great Spirit" sent "starberries" to ward off hunger and disease during a great famine. The United States and Canada are the largest producers and consumers of blueberries accounting for nearly 90% of the world's production. New Jersey, Michigan, North Carolina, and Oregon are the primary growing areas in the US.

Serving size is 1 cup (140 grams, 5 ounces). A serving contains 100 calories, 1 gram total fat, no saturated fat or cholesterol or sodium, 27 grams total carbohydrate (9% DV), 3 grams dietary fiber (14% DV), 11 grams sugars, 1 gram protein, 15% DV vitamin C, and 2% DV iron and folate.

Researchers at the USDA Human Nutrition Center report that blueberries rank among the highest in antioxidant activity when compared to 40 other fresh fruits and vegetables. Anthocyanin, the pigment that makes blueberries blue, is believed to play a major role in this antioxidant activity.

Blueberries contain a number of antioxidants. Chief among these include:

- beta carotene
- vitamins A and E
- phenolic compounds
- anthocyanins
- ellagic acid
- resveratrol

Owing to their high antioxidant activity, blueberries are reported to:

- slow age related loss in mental capacity

- have a beneficial effect on motor behavioral learning and memory

- improve eyesight and memory in the elderly

- reduce the build up of LDL cholesterol and help prevent cardiovascular disease and stroke

- reduce risk of certain types of cancer

- promote urinary tract health by preventing bacteria from adhering to the cells that line the walls of the urinary tract much in the same way as cranberries

While a great deal of interest is centered on the health benefits of red wine, blueberries appear to provide essentially the same basic phytonutrient compounds (anthrocyanins, flavonoids, and resveratrol). The latest interest in blueberries appears to be in resveratrol (3,5,4 trihydroxystilbene), a flavonoid and phytoestrogen. Resveratrol has been demonstrated not only to be a potent antioxidant (about 20-50 times more effective than vitamin C) but also to act synergistically with vitamin C, enhancing the effects of each. It also has been demonstrated to have an anticlotting effect that prevents the formation of thrombi (blood clots) that may block blood vessels and cause heart attacks and stroke. Also, resveratrol has shown significant anticancer effects and may delay the aging process.

Although their modes of action remain to be fully elucidated both ellagic and folic acids found in blueberries may inhibit cancer initiation. Ellagic acid (in its biologically active form, ellagitannin) has been shown to have significant anticancer activity. Folic acid may help guard against cervical cancer.

In Sweden, childhood diarrhea is treated with dried blueberries. Utility in this indication is believed to be due to anthocyanins inhibition E. coli bacteria linked to this infectious diarrhea.

Additional information on blueberries, history, nutrition content, research findings, health benefits, and recipes are available at:
http://www.ushbc.org/blueberry.htm
http://www ars.usda.gov (search "blueberries)

4.4.5.4 Cranberries

The cranberry plant is reported to have been in existence since the Iron Age. Romans are credited as the first to recognize the medicinal uses of cranberries. Currently there are around 150 species of cranberries in the world. The best known and most popular one is the American cranberry, vaccinium macrocarpon, because of its size and juiciness of its fruit. The US produces about 98% of the world's cranberries.

Serving size is 1 cup chopped raw cranberries (110 grams). A serving has around 54 calories, 0.4 gram of protein, 0.2 gram total fat, 14 grams of carbohydrate, 4.6 grams dietary fiber, 8 milligrams calcium, 78 milligrams of potassium, 15 milligrams of vitamin C, 56 I.U. vitamin A, 1 milligram sodium, and no cholesterol. Early sailing ships supplied their sailors with cranberries to prevent scurvy. The amount of vitamin C in one cup of raw cranberries is about one fourth of the current RDA for an adult. Cranberries also are considered to be a good source of dietary fiber and potassium.

Cranberries also are a rich source of phytonutrients with disease preventive properties including:

- anthocyanins and proanthocyanidins, compounds that prevent bacterial colonization/infection of the urinary tract and bladder

- antioxidants; cranberries are reported to contain more antioxidant compounds than 10 other commonly eaten fruits, and this may help protect against cardiovascular disease, cancer and other chronic disorders

- organic acids; including quinic, malic, and citric responsible for the sour taste and acidification of the urine and prevention of kidney stones

- a high molecular weight, nondializable substance that is reported to block adhesion of oral bacteria responsible for dental plaque and periodontal disease. Also, this substance is reported to inhibit the adhesion of Helicobacter pyloris in vitro, and may be active in preventing gastric cancer.

Studies suggest that diets containing fruits and vegetables with high antioxidant ORAC values (Oxygen Radical Absorbance Capacity) such as cranberries also may provide protection against age related problems of motor and cognitive function losses. Cranberries score among the highest of the fruits and vegetables in antioxidant ORAC values.

Additional cranberry information, nutritional content, selection, storage, preparation, and recipes are available at:
http://www.umext.maine.edu/onlinepubs/htmpubs/4308.htm
http://www.cranberrieinstitute.org/healthresearch.htm

4.4.5.5 Raspberries

The raspberry, Rubus idaeus, is regarded as indigenous to both Asia Minor and North America. Domestication of the red raspberry plant apparently took place in what is now Italy in the 4th century, according to Palladius, a Roman agriculturist. The Romans spread cultivation of the red raspberry plant throughout their empire, and raspberry seeds have been discovered in old Roman forts in Britain. King Edward I (1272-1307) apparently was the first person to favor cultivation of raspberries in Britain, and by the 18th century, raspberry cultivation had spread throughout Europe. First European settlers in America found Native Americans already consuming raspberries. However, it was not until 1771, that the first commercial raspberry plants were sold in America. By 1867, over 40 different varieties of red raspberries were known and cultivated in America.

Serving size is 1 cup (125 grams, 4.5 ounces). A serving contains around 50 calories, no fat or cholesterol or sodium, 17 grams total carbohydrates, 8 grams dietary fiber, 12 grams sugars, 1 gram protein, 40% DV Vitamin C, and 2% DV calcium and iron.

Men eating black raspberries consume the equivalent of around 12 milligrams of the phytonutrient, quercetin, per serving. Overall potential health benefits associated with quercetin include reduced risk of cancer, cardiovascular disease and cataracts as well as allergic and inflammatory disorders.

In addition to quercetin, black raspberries are reported to have the highest amount of another important phytonutrient, ellagic acid, an antioxidant that stimulates enzymes in the body to detoxify carcinogens, cancer producing substances. In animals, ellagic acid has been shown to have protective effects against esophageal and colon cancers.

Red raspberries also contain ellagic acid, a phenolic antioxidant phytonutrient and member of the ellagitannin family, which has become recognized as a potent anticarcinogenic and antimutagenic compound. Strawberries, pomegranates, and walnuts are reported to contain lesser amounts of this phytonutrient. However, ellagic acid is not believed to exist naturally by itself in red raspberries. Instead polymers of gallic acid and hexahydroxydipenoyl are linked to glucose to form the class of compounds known as ellagitannins in red raspberries. These phytonutrients are reported to:

- slow the growth of abnormal cells in the colon

- prevent the development of cells infected with the human papiloma virus linked to cervical cancer

- promote apoptotic death of prostate, breast, esophageal, lung, and skin cancer (melanoma) cells

- bind and inactivate cancer causing chemicals (carcinogens)

- inhibit chemicals causing mutations in bacteria

- prevent binding of carcinogens to DNA and reduce the incidence of cancer in cultured human cells exposed to carcinogens

Anthocyanins give black raspberries their color and are reported to have anti-inflammatory properties. Some cancers such as esophageal cancer have been linked to chronic inflammation, and further evaluation of anthocyanins in this disorder is indicated.

Additional information on raspberries and ellagic acid is available at:
http://www.ellagic-research.org/summary.htm
http://www.oregon-berries.com
http://www.cancer.org (search "ellagic acid")

4.4.5.6 Strawberries

The history of the strawberry dates back well over 2,000 years ago. In ancient Greek and Roman times, the strawberry was a wild plant. Its delicate heart shape became the symbol of Venus, the Goddess of Love. Strawberries were discovered in Virginia around 1600. Early settlers in Massachusetts enjoyed strawberries grown by local American Indians who mixed crushed strawberries with cornmeal and baked the mixture into a bread. The Colonists liked the strawberry bread so much that they developed their own version, and Strawberry Shortcake was born. California now produces 80% or more of the US consumption of strawberries. Strawberries are the only fruit with seeds on the outside rather than inside of the fruit.

Serving size is 8 medium strawberries (147 grams). A serving contains 0.5 gram total fat, no saturated fat or cholesterol or sodium, 17 grams carbohydrate (6% DV), 3.8 grams dietary fiber (8% DV), 8 grams sugars, 1 gram protein, 150% DV vitamin C (94 milligrams) and 2% DV calcium and iron. A serving of strawberries contains more vitamin C than an orange as well as 30 micrograms of folic acid and 275 milligrams of potassium.

Heart healthy substances in strawberries include vitamin C, potassium, folate, and antioxidant phytonutrients such as ellagic acid, quercetin, kaempferol, and phenolic acids. Vitamin C intake is correlated with a lower prevalence and death rate from cardiovascular disease (CVD) and reduced risk of angina. Folate reduces serum levels of homocysteine, a substance that is regarded as an independent risk factor for CVD (even a small elevation of homocysteine is estimated to increase CVD by 60% in men and 50% in women).

Research has demonstrated that individual phytonutirents in strawberries may have significant anticancer properties. Cancers of the colon, stomach, rectum, esophagus, lung, and pharynx as well as cancers of the breast, bladder, pancreas and larynx are among those that may be prevented by diets high in fruits and vegetables.

Strawberries have high total antioxidant activity. Ounce for ounce strawberries are reported to have 1.5 times more antioxidant activity than oranges and red grapes, 7 times more than apples, bananas, and tomatoes, 3 times more than kiwifruit or pink or white grapefruit, and 15 times more than pears and honeydew melons. Flavonoids (polyphenols) in strawberries with high antioxidant activity include anthocyanins, ellagic acid, kaempferol, and quercetin. Vitamin C also adds to the total antioxidant activity of strawberries. Antioxidants are believed to protect cells from free radical damage and cancer causing agents in at least two basic ways by blocking the initiation of carcinogenesis and suppressing its progression.

Chemically induced cancers of the esophagus, liver, lung, and skin are reported to be inhibited by ellagic acid. Quercetin also has been found to inhibit chemically induced cancers as well as the growth of human prostate and breast cancer cells in vitro. And, anthocyanins are reported to suppress the growth of colon cancer cells.

Epidemiologic research has provided further evidence that vitamin C reduces the risk for non hormone dependent cancers. Studies have demonstrated that vitamin C intake is associated with a reduction in the risk of breast and cervical cancers. Folate has been linked with a reduced risk for breast cancer in women who consume alcohol. Low folate intake may enhance the predisposition to cervical cancer in patients who are at increased risk due to papillomavirus exposure. Also, there is a relationship between low folate intake and the risk of colon cancer particularly in women over 50. Strawberries contain around 30 micrograms of folate per serving which can help offset low folate intake risks in women.

Additional information on the health benefits of strawberries is available at: http://www.calstrawberry.com/health/factsheet.asp

4.4.6 Broccoli

The word, broccoli comes from the Latin word brachium, which means branch or arm. Broccoli was first grown in the Italian province of Calabria. The most common type available today is the Italian green or sprouting variety.

Serving size is 3.5 ounces raw (1 cup chopped). One serving provides 28 calories with zero calories from fat, 10% DV for fiber, 30-40% DV for vitamin A, 155% DV for vitamin C, and 39% DV for folate. Broccoli is considered to be a good source of vitamins A and C, potassium, folate, iron and fiber. It has as much calcium per ounce as milk and contains a few important phytonutirents such as beta carotene, indoles, and isothiocynates. These phytonutrients may prevent carcinogens (cancer causing substances) from forming, or entering target cells, and help boost enzymes that detoxify carcinogens.

Recent studies have shown that frequent consumption of cruciferous vegetables is associated with a decreased risk for breast and colon cancer. High levels of the carotenoid lutein found in vegetables such as broccoli and spinach are associated with fewer cancers of the colon. Eating cruciferous vegetables also appears to reduce bladder cancer risk. In a study of 50,000 men, those who ate just two ½ cup servings of broccoli a week over a 10 year period had a 50% reduction in bladder cancer compared to men who rarely ate broccoli. Sulforaphane may be the primary cancer prevention agent in broccoli, and it is reported to reduce cancer development by 60 to 80% in laboratory animals. One ½ cup of broccoli sprouts is reported to have as much sulforaphane as 3-5 cups of broccoli. A related phytonutrient, indole-3-carbinol (13C) is reported to inhibit growth of cultured breast cancer cells.

Sulforaphane is also known as sulforaphane glucosinolate (SGS). Glucosinolates are primarily found in cruciferous vegetables (cabbage, broccoli, broccoli sprouts, brussels sprouts, cauliflower, cauliflower sprouts, bok choy, kale, collards, arugula, mustard, turnip, red radish, and watercress. Young broccoli and cauliflower sprouts are especially rich sources of these phytonutrients.

Sulforaphane is reported to significantly reduce the incidence of chemically induced mammary tumors in rats. It also has been shown to detoxify a number of carcinogens and thus may have the ability to protect against a variety of cancers. Dietary supplementation with sulforaphane enhances glutathione S-transferase (GST) enzyme activity, which is known to detoxify many carcinogens. Three day old sprouts of broccoli and cauliflower are reported to contain 10 to 100 times higher levels of glucoraphanin, the glucosinolate of sulforaphane, than do mature broccoli and cauliflower sprouts. Thus, small quantities of crucifer sprouts may more effectively protect against the risk of cancer.

Studies of sulforaphane (SGS) in human cell lines and laboratory animals provide evidence for its potential not only against cancer but also hypertension and macular degeneration, a leading cause of blindness in the elderly.

The dark green color in broccoli indicates high phytonutrient content. Florets (flower buds) that are dark green, purplish, or bluish green contain more beta carotene and vitamin C. Frozen broccoli has twice as much sodium, about half the calcium, and smaller amounts of iron, thiamine, riboflavin and vitamin C.

Make broccoli a part of a "5 to 9 a day" plan. Eat florets as a nutritious snack, eat them with a low fat dip, or include them in a salad. Include broccoli or another cruciferous vegetable in the dinner menu a few times a week.

Additional information on broccoli, selection, storage, fresh vs. frozen, preparation in cooking, inclusion in a "5 to 9 a day" plan, and recipes are available at:
http://www.cdc.gov/nccdphp/dnpa/5aday/month/broccoli.htm
http://www.cancer.org (search "broccoli and cancer")
http://www.brassica.com/press/pr00/2.htm

4.4.7 Brussels Sprouts

Brussels sprouts were named after the capital of Belgium, where it is thought that they were first cultivated. They look like miniature heads of cabbage, are similar in taste, and are slightly milder in flavor and denser in texture.

This vegetable contains significant amounts of vitamin C, beta carotene, and nitrogen containing compounds called indoles which may reduce the risk of certain cancers. They are also a good source of vegetable protein, because 31% of its calories come from protein. As the protein in brussel sprouts does not contain all essential amino acids and is incomplete, it should be consumed in meals with other protein sources that are complete such as meat or fish, for example.

Most brussels sprouts are grown in California and they are available all year round. Their peak growing season is autumn through early spring.

Serving size is ½ cup raw brussels sprouts (49 grams or 1-3/4 ounces). A serving contains 22 calories, no fat, low sodium, 195 milligrams potassium (10% DV), 1.5 grams of dietary fiber (7% DV), and 1.5 grams of protein.

Make brussels sprouts part of a "5 to 9 a day" plan. Blanched brussels sprouts make a great addition to salads, a nutritious snack, or an integral part of a vegetable tray. They have a hearty flavor, and go well with flavorful foods such as beef, sharp cheeses, or with stronger, seasoned foods, and make a tasty addition to soups, stews and casseroles.

Additional information on brussel sprouts, selection, storage, preparation, inclusion in a "5 to 9 a day" plan and recipes are available at: http://www.cdc.gov/nccdphp/dnpa/5aday/month/sprouts.htm

4.4.8 Cabbage

Cabbage is one of the oldest vegetables and an inexpensive dietary staple. There are at least 100 different types of cabbage grown throughout the world with the green, red and Savoy varieties being the most commonly consumed in the United States. The two most common types of Chinese cabbage are Bok Choy and Napa cabbage that cook in less time than standards US types.

Serving size is 3.5 ounces of raw cabbage (1.5 cups shredded). One serving has 33 calories and is considered to be rich in vitamin C (47% DV), moderate in vitamin A (15% DV), reasonably good in dietary fiber (2 grams or 8% DV), and low in sodium, potassium and protein. Cabbage has no fat.

Cabbage should be part of a "5 to 9 a day" plan. It can be steamed, boiled, microwaved, stuffed, or stir fried. Cut up fresh cabbage, sprinkle with lemon and enjoy it as a midday snack. Include cabbage in a salad. Try adding cabbage to vegetable soup or as a cooked vegetable with a meal (e.g. corned beef and cabbage).

Individuals who frequently consume cabbage and other cruciferous vegetables in their diet may help to reduce their risk of certain cancers such as colon and rectal cancer. This may be due to the action of sulfur containing compounds.

Precut cabbage easily loses significant vitamin C content. Keep cabbage cold and in a plastic bag and store in the refrigerator to preserve its vitamin C content.

Fermenting cabbage into sauerkraut is reported to release isothiocynates, phytonutrients also thought to be protective against cancer.

Additional information on cabbage varieties, selection, storage, preparation, and recipes are available at:
http://www.cdc.gov/nccdphp/dnpa/5aday/month/cabbage.htm

4.4.9 Carrots

Carrots may be referred to as "good for the eyes". However, carrots are rich in vitamin A that is important not only for healthy eyesight but also for skin health, growth and development, and resistance to infection.

There are many varieties of carrots. The one typically found in supermarkets is from 7-9 inches in length and ¾ to 1.5 inches in diameter. Baby carrots are ones that have been peeled, trimmed to 1.5 inches in length, narrowed in diameter and washed and packaged.

Serving size is equivalent to one 6-7 inch long, 1.5 inch in diameter carrot (78 grams). One serving contains around 35 calories, no cholesterol or fat, 1 gram protein and is low in sodium (25 milligrams). It also contains vitamin A (270% DV), vitamin C (10% DV), and 2 grams of dietary fiber (8% DV).

Carrots are easily incorporated into a "5 to 9 a day" plan. Raw carrots can be used as a snack between meals, at lunch, or at a picnic, as well as "on the go". Carrots can be eaten raw, cut into sticks or rounds, and chopped or shredded into salads. They have a higher natural sugar content than all other vegetables with the exception of beets. This may be one reason why they make a wonderful snack when eaten raw, or as a tasty addition to a variety of cooked dishes.

Carrots are considered an excellent source of the carotenoid, beta carotene linked to reducing chronic diseases such as cancer, cardiovascular disease, etc. Eating carrots may also lower blood cholesterol levels. Women who ate just 4 carrot sticks at least 5 days a week are reported to have reduced their risk of ovarian cancer, the fifth deadliest cancer in women, by 50%.

Additional carrot information, varieties, selection, storage, preparation, inclusion in a "5 to 9 a day" plan, and recipes are available at: http://www.cdc.gov/nccdphp/dnpa/5aday/month/carrots.htm

4.4.10 Cauliflower

Cauliflower is a cruciferous vegetable. In its early stages, it resembles broccoli, its closest relative. While broccoli opens outward to sprout bunches of green florets, cauliflower forms a compact head of undeveloped flower buds with green leaves surrounding the head to protect the flower buds from sunlight. Lack of exposure to sunlight does not allow chlorophyll to develop, therefore, color is not produced, and the head remains white in color. There are two common types of cauliflower on the market in the US today. The creamy white florets are more common but a recently developed cauliflower broccoli hybrid has a green head and resembles broccoli. The green variety is less dense, cooks more quickly and has a milder taste.

Serving size is 1/6 medium cauliflower (99 grams/3.5 ounces) One serving contains around 100% of the DV for vitamin C, 200 milligrams potassium (8% DV), and 2 grams dietary fiber (8% DV). It is low in sodium and contains little or no fat or cholesterol.

Cauliflower is easily incorporated into a "5 to 9 a day" plan. Raw florets make a crunchy, nutritious appetizer with a low fat dressing or dip. Fresh or leftover cauliflower can be added to soups or stews. Chopped florets can be used in place of meatballs as a addition to pasta sauce for a vegetarian pasta dish, and also as an addition to a tossed salad. It also may be substituted for broccoli in a number of dishes. Cooked cauliflower may be stirred into mashed potatoes to enhance their texture.

Currently, cauliflower is being evaluated for its possible role in reducing cancer risk.

Additional cauliflower information, varieties, selection, storage, preparation, inclusion in a "5 to 9 a day" plan, and recipes are available at: http://www.cdc.gov/nccdphp/dnpa/5aday/month/cauliflower.htm

4.4.11 Celery

Celery is derived from wild celery thought to have originated in the Mediterranean regions of northern Africa and southern Europe as well as East Asia. It apparently was first used as a medicine and then later as a food. Knowledge of the medicinal properties of celery leaves dates back to the 9th century BC, being mentioned in the *Odyssey* by the Greek poet, Homer. Early varieties of celery differed somewhat from its modern day counterpart, having less stalks and more leaves. Ancient Greeks used celery leaves as laurels to decorate renowned athletes, while the Romans used it principally as a seasoning, a tradition that has carried through the centuries. Celery is regarded as a common household staple along with carrots, onions and potatoes. Although it is available throughout the year, the best tasting celery is found during the summer months when it is in season. It grows to a height of 12-16 inches, and is a member of the Umbelliferae family whose other members include carrots, fennel, and parsley.

Serving size is 1 cup of raw, chopped celery or 2 medium stalks (110 grams). A serving contains 20 calories, 12-15% DV vitamin C, 8-12% DV potassium, molybdenum, folate, vitamin B-6 (pyrodoxine), manganese, and dietary fiber as well as 4-6% DV calcium and 2% DV iron. It contains no fat, 100 milligrams sodium, 2% DV carbohydrate, 3 grams sugars, 1 gram protein, and 2% DV vitamin A. The leaves contain most of the celery's nutritional benefits.

In addition to vitamin C, celery contains disease preventive phytonutrients that promote health. Its vitamin C may help protect against certain chronic diseases, particularly age related disorders, cancer, heart disease and stroke. Celery contains, in addition to good amounts of potassium, a pthalide compound (3-n-butylphthalide) that dilates blood vessels and regulates blood pressure. Blood pressure may be lowered some 12-14% in animals with a dose equivalent to around 4 stalks of celery in humans. Pthalides also reduce stress hormone levels (catecholamines) which causes blood vessels to constrict, elevating blood pressure.

In addition, celery has been shown in animals to lower blood cholesterol, have a diuretic activity, and prevent cancer. Celery's phytonutrient coumarins help prevent free radicals from damaging cells, thus decreasing mutations and the potential for cells to become cancerous. Other phytonutrients in celery, called aceylenics, have been shown to stop the growth of tumor cells. And, phenolic acids in celery have been shown to block the actions of prostaglandins known to encourage the growth of cancerous cells.

Celery is easily incorporated into a "5 to 9 a day" plan. Add chopped celery to a favorite tuna fish dish or salad, or chicken salad recipe. Enjoy the traditional peanut better spread on celery stalks as a snack. Use celery leaves or chopped celery in salads. Add celery leaves or slice stalks into soups, stews, casseroles, and healthy stir-fry.

Additional celery information, history, health benefits, nutritional profile, selection, storage, and recipes are available at:
http://www.whfoods.com/genpage.
php?tname=foodspice&dbid=14healthbenefits
http://www.personalhealthzone.
com/nutrition/nutrients/vegetables/celery.html

4.4.12 Cherries

Cherries are believed to have originated in Asia and were subsequently dispersed throughout Europe and North America in ancient times. European colonists found wild cherry trees in America when they first arrived and crossbred them with European varieties. As the popularity and nutritional value of cherries grew throughout the world over the years, the United States became the world leader among the top 20 producing countries. Now, some 70% of all cherries produced in the US come from 4 states, namely Washington, Oregon, Idaho and Utah.

Basically, there are two varieties of cherries, the sweet and the sour. Sweets are further categorized by color, dark and light skinned. Of the dark skinned variety, the "Bing is king". Royal Annes, also called Raniers, are amber to yellow in color with a red blush, and the more common variety among the light skinned. Sour cherries are bright scarlet in color and are mostly canned or frozen and used in pie fillings or sauces.

Sweet cherries
Serving size for the sweet cheery is one cup (pitted). A serving contains 104 calories, 1.4 grams total fat, 0.3 gram saturated fat, and the rest unsaturated fat, 3.3 grams dietary fiber, 2 grams protein, 1.1 milligrams beta carotene, and 16 milligrams vitamin C.

Sour cherries
Serving size for the sour cherry is 1 cup (pitted). A serving contains 78 calories, 0.5 gram total fat, 0.1 gram saturated fat, and the rest unsaturated fat, 2.5 grams dietary fiber, 2 grams of protein, 1.1 milligrams of beta carotene, and 16 milligrams of vitamin C.

Cherries are juicy, tasty, colorful and have significant nutrient content in the form of vitamin C, beta carotene, potassium (270 milligrams) and pectin (a soluble fiber). They also are reported to be high in disease preventive phytonutrients such as:

- anthocyanins that may provide defense against cancer causing carcinogens. Cherries have a high ORAC (antioxidant) score that appears to be correlated with their anthocyanin content.

- quercetin that appears to have not only anticancer properties but also anti-inflammatory and antihistamine activity as well.

- melatonin, a potent antioxidant regarded as more potent in this regard than vitamin C, E, and A due to its water solubility and ability to more easily enter certain cells. Cherry juice concentrate is reported to have ten times the melatonin content compared to the raw fresh fruit. Melatonin is also a potential sleep enhancer. About 3.5 ounces (100 grams) of tart cherries contains around 27 milligrams of melatonin compared with only 7 milligrams in sweet cherries.

- phenols which account for much of the total antioxidant activity

- ellagic acid, a phenolic compound that is reported to be cancer preventive.

- perillyl alcohol, a monoterpene alcohol reported to have significant anticancer activity. Monoterpenes are found in the essential oils of cherries. Perillyl alcohol is reported to be active against human pancreatic, colon, and liver cancers, and preventive against colon, prostate, lung, and ultraviolet light induced skin cancer.

- beta sitosterol, a phytosterol linked to lower blood cholesterol levels

- a yet undefined substance that is reported to help prevent tooth decay.

Cherries can easily be incorporated into a "5 to 9 day" plan by:

- serving them fresh as a snack or for dessert

- poaching and serving them with a meal

- sautéing and serving them in crepes, atop pancakes or waffles, or over frozen yogurt

- cooking them in pies

- making them into jams and preserves

- drinking cherry juice

Additional cherries information, varieties, storage, preparation, inclusion in a "5 to 9 a day" plan, and recipes are available at:
http://www.nwcherries.com/health.html

4.4.13 Corn

Corn has been an important nutritional resource for thousands of years because of its high protein and carbohydrate content. It can be traced back to Central American cultures as early as 3,400 BC. Americans consume about 25 pounds of corn per person annually most of which is frozen or canned, both having about the same nutritional value as fresh corn. There are more than 200 varieties of corn. All are considered to be good sources of vitamin C but only yellow kernels contain small amounts of vitamin A in the form of beta carotene.

Serving size is one medium ear of corn (99 grams/3.2 ounces). A serving contains 80 calories, 1 gram of unsaturated fat, no cholesterol, 240 milligrams potassium (7% DV), 18 grams carbohydrate (6% DV), 3 grams dietary fiber (12%) DV), vitamin C (10% DV), small amounts of vitamin A (2% DV), and 3 grams of protein. Although corn is higher in protein content than any other vegetable, its protein is incomplete since it lacks the essential amino acids lysine and tryptophan. To create a complete protein content, with all the essential amino acids, corn should be consumed with legumes (beans, lentils, or split peas), fish or meat. Legumes contain high levels of lysine and tryptophan. By combining the two (a grain and a legume), a complete non animal source of protein is created.

According to Cornell University food scientists, cooking sweet corn, whether you cream it or steam it on the cob, releases beneficial phytonutrients that may substantially reduce the risk of cancer or cardiovascular disease. This finding contradicts previous held beliefs that processed fruits and vegetables have a lower nutritional value compared with fresh produce. In fact, research now indicates that cooked sweet corn, not only retains its antioxidant activity despite the loss of vitamin C but that the antioxidant activity is increased by cooking. Cooked sweet corn releases a phenolic compound called ferulic acid, bound to corn cell walls and insoluble fibers. Available ferulic acid is reported to be substantially increased after sweet corn was cooked at 115 degrees Celsius (239F) for 10, 25 and 50 minutes by 40%, 550% and 900% respectively.

Ferulic acid, a long known antioxidant phytochemical is found in very low amounts in fruits and vegetables, however, very high levels are reported to exist in corn. Generally, ferulic acid is found mostly in whole grains. In addition to ferulic acid, sweet corn also is considered to be high in phenolic antioxidants.

Corn is easy to incorporate into a "5 to 9 day" plan. Grilled or microwaved ears of corn are a tasty treat. Kernels of corn are a great addition when mixed with other vegetables. Corn may be added to a favorite vegetable soup, or in rice to add color, or in tossed salads.

Additional corn information, varieties, storage, inclusion in a "5 to 9 a day" plan and recipes are available at:
http://www.cdc.gov/nccdphp/dnpa/5aday/month/corn.htm
http://www.sciencedaily.com/releases/2002/08/020812070350.htm

4.4.14 Dried Beans

From the royal tombs of ancient Egypt to the Old Testament and on to Western civilization, beans have been recognized as a good nutrition source. The United States is the world's leader in dry bean production, totaling some 1.5 to 1.7 million acres of edible dry beans grown annually, with around 40% being shipped to international markets in over 100 countries.

Serving size is 1/3 cup of cooked beans. In general, one serving contains around 80 calories, no fat or cholesterol, and mostly complex carbohydrate. In addition, beans are low in sodium and a good source of B vitamins (e.g., folate), potassium, iron, and fiber. The fiber content tends to promote better health and relieves constipation. There are hundreds of varieties of beans and the nutrient content of each varies.

Dried beans are an inexpensive and healthy inclusion in a "5 to 9 a day" plan. While beans may be served as a side dish, they make excellent meat free entrees. However, don't just limit beans to entree dishes, use them in soups, for dips, and in salads. Substitute beans for a meatless meal 1-2 times a week. In any event, be sure to serve beans with vitamin C rich vegetables in a meal to aid in the absorption of the iron in the beans.

It is important to recognize that the protein in dried beans is not a complete protein since it does not contain all the essential amino acids in recommended amounts. So it is essential that beans be consumed with whole grain products (e.g. beans and whole grain rice, split pea soup, or corn bread) that do contain necessary complete protein sources.

Legumes may cause intestinal discomfort in some individuals. This can be minimized by changing the soaking water several times when dried beans are prepared, or by switching to canned beans which eliminates some of the gas producing substances. Another option is to use the product "Beano" which contains an enzyme that breaks down gas producing substances (oligosaccharides) in beans. As more beans are included in meals, it is important to drink adequate fluids and exercise regularly so the gastrointestinal system can handle the increased dietary fiber.

Additional dried bean information, varieties, nutrient profiles, preparation, cooking, inclusion in a "5 to 9 a day" plan, and recipes are available at: http://www.cdc.gov/nccdphp/dnpa/5aday/month/beans.htm

4.4.15 Figs

Figs have provided dietary sustenance since ancient times. Both fresh and dried figs have been favored historically. While figs originally came from sunny spots around the Mediterranean, today's figs consumed in the US originate from California's San Joaquin Valley. California now ranks number two in the world in fig production. Figs are regarded as an important dietary food source because they are nutritious, nutrient dense, portable, versatile and tasty, meet the needs of today's lifestyles, and contain important disease preventative polyphenol phytonutrients.

One serving of figs is 40 grams or about ¼ cup or 3 Calimyra figs or 4 to 5 Mission figs, and contains about 113 calories. Figs are low in fat, sodium free, and like other plant foods, cholesterol free. A serving is high in dietary fiber having around 5 grams or 20% of the DV, more fiber per serving than any other common dried or fresh fruit. Four grams of this fiber are insoluble and one gram is water soluble. Also contained in one serving are 244 milligrams of potassium (7% DV), 53 milligrams of calcium (6% DV), 1.2 milligrams of iron (6% DV), 26 grams of carbohydrate and 1.3 grams of protein.

Figs fit nicely into a "5 to 9 a day" plan. Use them as a snack at home, in the office, or at a picnic. Slice a few figs to add to a tossed salad for sweetness, texture, and fiber. Sweeten up mashed or cubed squash or sweet potatoes with chopped figs. Blend low fat ricotta or cottage cheese with figs to create a tasty spread for toast or bagels, or as a dip. Scatter chopped figs over cereal for breakfast or enjoy some for lunch. Choosing figs and other high fiber foods more frequently may reduce consumption of less healthy foods.

Dried figs are reported to have a polyphenol, antioxidant compound content ranging from 4 to 50 times higher than most other fruits. To put this data in perspective, 100 grams of processed California dried figs provide more polyphenol content than the total daily per capita consumption of polyphenols from 21 commonly consumed vegetables or fruits. Dried figs also are reported to contain omega-3 and omega-6 fatty acids as well as a number of phytosterols.

Additional fig information, history, nutritional content and recipes are available at:
http://www.californiafigs.com
http://www.californiafigs.com/nutrition/index.html

4.4.16 Grapefruit

Grapefruit, as we know it today, originated in the West Indies and was introduced to Florida in the 1820s. Today, most grapefruit consumed in the US is still grown in Florida. It was named by the way it grows in clusters, like grapes, on a tree. There are three major types of grapefruit, white, pink/red, and star ruby/rio red. All grapefruits have a similar tangy sweet flavor and are juicy. The pink or red varieties contain more vitamins and phytonutrients.

Serving size is ½ of a medium grapefruit (154 grams). A serving contains around 60 calories, including 10 grams of sugars. Grapefruits are considered to be rich in vitamin C (115% DV) and dietary fiber (6 grams or 24% DV), and contain some vitamin A (15% DV).

Grapefruit is easily included in a "5 to 9 a day" plan. Half a grapefruit may be eaten in the morning with cereal. A small can of grapefruit juice may be consumed at lunch instead of soda pop. Peeled segments of grapefruit may be included in salads or eaten with a dash of cinnamon as a snack.

Grapefruit juice may interfere with medications being taken, significantly increasing blood levels and adverse reactions. Some medications reported to be affected in this way include cyclosporin (Sandimmune, Neoral), lovastatin (Mevacor), midazolam (Versed), pravastatin (Pravachol), and thyroid medications. Certain antihistamines such as astemizol (Hismanal) and terfenadine (Seldane and Seldane D) may have increased drug levels associated with cardiac arrhythmias that may be fatal.

If grapefruit, or its juice is consumed regularly and medication is being taken, a physician needs to be consulted for the appropriate course of action to take.

Additional grapefruit information, varieties, storing, nutritive values, inclusion in a "5 to 9 a day" plan, and recipes are available at:
http://www.cdc.gov/nccdphp/dnpa/5aday/month/grapefruit.htm

4.4.17 Grapes/Raisins/Grape Juice/Wine

4.4.17.1 Grapes

Grapes are one of the oldest dietary fruits to be cultivated. Spanish explorers introduced the fruit to America, and grapes are now grown in a number of states. The Old World or wine grape is Vitis vinifera, the purple Concord and similar varieties are Vitis labrusca. Grapes come in more than 50 varieties and colors. Two main type of grapes are American and European. They both come in seeded and seedless varieties, and most are grown in California. Concord grapes are considered to be excellent for table use and for making juice and jelly. The larger, purplish red Catawba variety is used primarily for juice and wine. Both can be served fresh for eating.

Serving size is 1.5 cups of grapes (138 grams). One serving contains 90 calories, 1 gram of fat, no sodium, 270 milligrams potassium (8% DV), 20 grams carbohydrate (7% DV), 1 gram fiber, 1 gram protein, and vitamin C (25% DV). Grapes are 80% water.

Grapes contain resveratrol, quercetin, anthocyanins, and catechins, all powerful antioxidant compounds. These phytonutrients are reported to inhibit the development of some types of cancer, protect against cardiovascular disease, and may also be useful in the prevention of other conditions such as arthritis, allergies, circulatory problems, diabetes, and age related macular degeneration and cataracts. Resveratrol, found chiefly in the skin of red/purple grapes, is now being evaluated mainly for the prevention of cardiovascular disease and cancer, and antiaging effects

Grapes are easily included in a "5 to 9 a day" plan. A cup of Concord or Catawba grapes makes a delectable low calorie, low fat snack or dessert. Grapes may be added to any meal as a side dish. They can be frozen, eaten for breakfast with whole grain cereal or lunch. They are the original fast food.

Whole grapes have been associated with health for many centuries now. However, exclusive grape diets like the ones promoted by Dr. Johanna Brandt, in the early 1900s at the Harmony Healing Center in New York City, or Dr. Harvey Kellogg, the corn flake king at his clinic in Battlecreek, Michigan, are no longer recommended.

Additional information on grapes, varieties, selection, using and preserving grapes, inclusion in a "5 to 9 a day" plan and recipes are available at: http://www.cdc.gov/nccdphp/dnpa/5aday/month/grapes.htm http://www.tablegrape.com/health/phytochem.asp

4.4.17.2 Raisins

Raisins are believed to date back to around 1500 BC. Muscat, oversized raisins with tiny seeds, were grown in Southern Spain, and farmers in Greece grew tiny seedless, tangy raisins called currants. Crusader knights introduced raisins to Europe and they became an important part of European cuisine. In the 18th century, Spanish missionaries helped farmers in California grow grapes for wine and a marketable muscat for raisins in the 1850s. Around 1876, a Scottish immigrant, William Thompson, grew a seedless grape variety that was thin skinned, seedless, sweet and tasty. Today 95 % of California raisins are made from Thompson seedless grapes.

Serving size is ¼ cup raisins (40 grams). A serving contains 130 calories, no fat, 10 milligrams of sodium, 310 milligrams potassium (9% DV), 31 grams total carbohydrate (10% DV), 2 grams dietary fiber (8% DV), 29 grams sugars, 1 gram protein, less than 2% DV for vitamins A and C, 2% DV calcium, and

6% DV iron. Per serving, raisins are higher in calories (130 vs. 90), grams of carbohydrate (31 vs. 20), milligrams of potassium (310 vs. 270), grams dietary fiber (2 vs. 1) but lower in grams of total fat (0 vs. 1), vitamin C (less than 2% vs. 25%) and water (a little vs. 80%) compared with a serving of grapes. The phytonutrient content and health benefits of raisins are believed to be similar to grapes.

Raisins can easily be incorporate into a "5 to 9 a day" plan by eating them as a snack alone or with nuts, using them in baked goods (e.g. muffins) or as a topping on cereal, incorporating them in sauces, stews, desserts and salads, or employing ¼ cup as one sweet, delicious serving of fruit

Additional information about raisins, history, nutrition, health benefits and recipes are available at:
http://www.calraisins.org

4.4.17.3 Grape Juice

For those who do not like wine, purple grape juice provides almost the same, but not quite all, the potential health benefits that may be obtained from red wine. Grape juice is reported to contain essentially the same phytonutrient antioxidants, that are believed to give red wine many of its disease preventive benefits. Flavonoids (polyphenols) in grape juice are reported to reduce low density lipoprotein (LDL) oxidation and improve blood circulation. In addition, grape juice appears to provide the health benefits without the potential deleterious effects, of alcohol. However, red wine, due to its alcohol content, raises HDL, high density lipoprotein levels in blood, which is regarded as cardioprotective, whereas purple grape juice does not.

4.4.17.4 Wine

The American Heart Association (AHA) recommends that if you drink wine, do so in moderation. This means an average of one to two drinks per day for men, and one drink per day for women. A drink is limited to 4 ounces.

Drinking more than recommended levels of alcohol may:

• raise levels of some fats in the blood such as triglycerides

- lead to high blood pressure, stroke, cardiomyopathy, cardiac arrhythmias, and sudden death

- produce excessive caloric intake, overweight and obesity

- increase the risk of developing diabetes mellitus

- increase the risk of breast cancer in women

- reduce life expectancy

Life expectancy falls with more than one drink a day for women and more than 2 drinks a day for men. Just 4-5 drinks within 24 hours, a common occurrence at social events, increases the short term risk of a stroke almost fivefold in those at high risk. Even one drink a day appears to increase a woman's risk of dying from breast cancer.

Moderate drinking, on the other hand, may reduce the risk of cardiovascular disease and is regarded as "heart healthy". Red wine may lower blood pressure, increase HDL-C, increase nitric oxide (NO) production that helps dilate blood vessels and prevent blood clotting, and reduce free radical damage via its antioxidant activity. However, AHA cautions individuals not to start drinking if they do not already drink alcohol without consulting their doctor regarding the benefit to risk ratio in consuming alcohol.

Red wine is a rich source of phytonutrients called flavonoids (polyphenols). They include catechin, epicatechin, gallic acid, and proanthocyanidins, and resveratrol. These are found chiefly in the skin and seeds of grapes. When wine is made, alcohol produced by the fermentation process dissolves the polyphenols contained in the skin and seeds. Red wine contains more polyphenols than white wine because the making of white wine requires the removal of the skins after the grapes are crushed. Among the red wines, cabernet sauvignon and pinot noir are reported to have the most polyphenols, and merlots and red zinfandels somewhat fewer.

Polyphenols are antioxidant compounds that protect cells from oxidative damage caused by free radicals. Cellular damage caused by free radicals has been implicated in the development of cancer and cardiovascular disease. Antioxidants found in red wine also have been shown to inhibit the three stages in the cancer process: initiation, promotion, and progression.

Resveratrol, (trihydroxystilbene), is a type of polyphenol. A fluid ounce of red wine contains approximately 160 micrograms of resveratrol, compared to peanuts, which average around 73 micrograms per ounce. Resveratrol has been shown to reduce tumor incidence in animals and inhibit cancer cells in culture, and reduce inflammation. However, resveratrol appears to be a less effective antioxidant compared with quercetin and epicatechin, also found in red wine and may not be the whole answer. Also, recommending a population wide increase in red wine may be premature at this time because:

- levels of flavonoids appear to vary widely in various red wine products

- not enough is known about the flavonoids contained in red wine and their utility in preventing cancer and cardiovascular disease

- the role of resveratrol as a phytoestrogen and possible potentiator of breast cancinomas may limit its use

- recommending increased consumption of red wine to boost resveratrol intake may due more harm than good

Additional information on the potential health benefits of wine and its phyto-nutrient ingredients are available at:
http://www.nlm.nih.gov/medlineplus (search "wine")
http://www.cdc.gov/od/ohs/vitamin/928.htm
http://www.cancer.gov/newscenter/pressreleases/redwine

4.4.18 Kiwis

The kiwifruit is around 700 years old, originating in the Yangtse river valley in China where it was called "Yangtao". Seeds were sent to New Zealand in 1906, and the fruit was renamed there the "Chinese gooseberry". New Zealand's "Chinese Gooseberry" variety was first brought to the United States in 1962 where it was renamed kiwifruit after New Zealand's native bird, the "kiwi". In the 1970s, kiwis were grown commercially in California for the first time, and became available in supermarkets here. Most kiwifruit imported into the United States comes from Chile and New Zealand and is available year-round. There are 400 or so varieties of kiwifruit. They may be trained to grown on a trellis with vines climbing up to 15 feet in height.

Serving size is 2 medium kiwis (148 grams). One serving contains 100 calories, 1 gram of fat, no cholesterol or sodium, 24 grams of carbohydrate, 4 grams of fiber, vitamin C (240% DV), 2 grams of protein, some calcium (6% DV), and iron (4% DV). Kiwis are regarded as a reasonably good source of vitamin E and potassium.

A lesser known fact about kiwis is that they contain a natural meat tenderizer, an enzyme called actinidin which helps digest protein. This enzyme also breaks down protein in dairy products. Therefore, when kiwi is combined with low fat ice cream, yogurt, or sour cream, it is best to serve and eat it right away.

Kiwi can easily be incorporated into a "5 to 9 a day" plan. Its skin is very thin and edible. Have a kiwi for a snack, cut it in half through the middle and scoop out each half with a spoon, and eat it. Peel and slice kiwi in a fruit salad or on breakfast cereal. Garnish lunch or dinner entrees with kiwi slices or wedges.

Additional kiwi information, varieties, storage, preparation, inclusion in a "5 to 9 a day" plan and recipes are available at:
http://www.cdc.gov/nccdphp/dnpa/5aday/month/kiwi.htm

4.4.19 Lemons

Lemons are reported to have originated in China, and lemonade may have been a favorite drink of the Chinese Emperors. Catholic missionaries are reported to have facilitated the lemon's entry into the United States, and its original planting in Arizona and California. Today, virtually all the lemons consumed in the US as well as about one third used throughout the world are produced by these two states. There are two different varieties of lemons, acid and sweet. Eurekas and Lisbons are the most common acid types grown commercially. Sweet lemon types are grown mainly by home gardeners. Lemon trees bloom continuously all year long and can produce up to 500 to 600 lemons a year each.

Serving size is 1 medium lemon (58 grams/2.1 ounces). One serving contains 15 calories, no fat, cholesterol or protein, 5 grams carbohydrate, 1 gram dietary fiber, 1 gram sugars, vitamin C (40% DV), and very little calcium. Lemons are regarded as a good source for vitamin C.

Lemons are valued chiefly for their many uses in flavoring the food we eat, as a garnish, and household purposes. They are easily incorporated into a "5 to 9 a day" plan. Use lemons in marinades, especially for chicken and fish. Sprinkle lemon juice on top of steamed vegetables, seafood and salads. Mix salad dressing with lemon instead of vinegar. Fresh grated lemon peels add zest to baked goods, fruit salads, desserts and sauces. Replace other fruits with lemon in frozen sorbet. Add lemon juice or a slice of fresh lemon to water in increase consumption of water during the day.

Lemon peel is a source of limonene, a phytonutrient being studied for its potential as an anticancer agent.

Additional lemon information, selection, storage, preparation, varieties, tips, inclusion in a "5 to 9 a day" plan and recipes are available at: http://www.cdc.gov/nccdphp/dnpa/5aday/month/lemon.htm

4.4.20 Lentils/Dried Peas/Chickpeas/Soybeans

4.4.20.1 Lentils

Lentils are related to beans and both are considered to be members of the legume family, seeds that grow within pods. The Latin word for lentil is lens, and lentils are shaped like a lens. A lentil's outer seed coat can be mottled or speckled, and have a color ranging from reddish brown to grayish brown to green. The inner coat, the cotyledon, can be yellow or red.

Serving size is ¼ cup (35 grams) boiled lentils. A serving contains 130 calories. Total fat is 0.5 grams, carbohydrates 22 grams (7% DV), dietary fiber 11 grams (44% DV), protein 8 grams, and iron (14% DV). There is no cholesterol, saturated fat, sugars, or sodium in a serving. Lentils are considered to be an excellent source of protein, fiber, complex carbohydrate, and folic acid, and they are a low calorie, low fat, and cholesterol free food as well as being inexpensive.

Folic acid is a very important nutrient found in lentils. One cup of cooked lentils provides 90% of the recommended daily allowance (RDA) of folic acid. As such, lentils provide more folic acid than any other unfortified food. While lentils are considered to be protein rich, lentil protein is incomplete, lacking only one essential amino acid, methionine. Consuming whole grains, eggs, meat, fish, or dairy products along with lentils supplies the necessary amount of the missing amino acid, methionine for completeness. Soluble fiber contained in lentils serves to decrease blood glucose and cholesterol levels, and may decrease medication requirements for individuals with diabetes mellitus.

4.4.20.2 Dried Peas

Dried peas originated in ancient times. Peas may be dried in the sun and split by bombarding them against a baffle. The split pea process decreases required cooking time.

Serving size is 1.4 cup (35 grams) cooked peas. A serving contains 130 calories, 0.5 gram total fat, and no saturated fat, cholesterol, sodium or sugars. Carbohydrate content is 23 grams (8% DV), dietary fiber 10 grams (40% DV), and protein 8 grams. Peas are considered to be a high protein food, and a good source for potassium and the B vitamins, especially folate. Carbohydrates are complex and release energy slowly.

One half cup of cooked peas or lentils provides more than 10 grams dietary fiber, and a high fiber diet may help prevent cardiovascular disease and some cancers. Folate content also may help prevent heart disease.

Americans generally are more familiar with fresh green peas, covered in section 4.4.29.

4.4.20.3 Chickpeas

Chickpeas originally were cultivated in the eastern Mediterranean and Mesopotamia areas in ancient times. They also are referred to as garbanzo beans and serve as rotation crops to wheat and barley, replenishing nitrogen to the soil and reducing the need for chemical fertilizers.

Serving size is ¼ cup (35 grams) cooked chickpeas. A serving contains 115 calories, 1.75 grams fat with no saturated fat or cholesterol. Carbohydrate content is 19 grams (7% DV), dietary fiber 11 grams (44% DV), protein 7 grams, and iron 12% DV. Chickpeas contain no sugars or sodium

Chickpeas as well as other legumes, being high in fiber, help decrease blood glucose and cholesterol levels and improve management of diabetes mellitus. Legumes, including chickpeas are an integral part of the popular Mediterranean diet.

Additional information, varieties, nutrition, preparation, and recipes for lentils, dried peas, and chickpeas are available at:
http://www.pea-lentil.com/kitchen.html
http://www.pea-lentil.com/nutrition.html

4.4.20.4 Soybeans

Emperor Ching Nung is reported to have provided the first written record of the soybean in 2838 BC. The ancient Chinese refered to a group of five sacred grains, as "Wu Ku"(soybean, rice, wheat, barley and millet) considered essential for the existence of the Chinese civilization. The soybean was domesticated in the eastern half of north China in the 11th century, and introduced into Korea and Japan between 200 BC and 300 AD. It was not until 1765 that the first soybean was planted in the United States in Georgia. Before 1898, only eight soybean varieties were known in the US, representing yellow, black, green and brown, seed coats. By 1910, the number had grown to 280 varieties, and today more than 2,500 varieties are cultivated throughout the world. The US soybean plant is an annual that has oblong pods that contain 2 to 4 seeds.

In the US the soybean generally is not consumed per se but usually is processed into a variety of products. Soy products are widely consumed in the US today. In fact, soybean oil accounts for around 80% of the edible fats consumed annually in the US (e.g., in commercial mayonnaise, margarine, salad dressing, or vegetable shortening). Soy protein products include such things as:

- tofu, made from cooked pureed soybean and processed into a custard cake, with firm, soft, and silken textures and a neutral flavor. Tofu can be stir fried, mixed into smoothies, or blended into a cream cheese texture for use in dips, or as a cheese substitute

- soy milk, a soy beverage produced by grinding dehulled beans and mixing them with water to form a milk like liquid. This can be consumed as a beverage or used in recipes as a substitute for cow's milk. It can be fortified with calcium and comes in vanilla, chocolate, or coffee flavors, and is a good replacement for milk for lactose intolerant individuals.

- soy flour, created by grinding roasted soybeans into a fine flour which can be added to baked goods in place of eggs. Soy flour also can be used in cereals, pancake mixes, frozen desserts, and other common foods.

- textured soy protein, made from defatted soy flour and compressed and dehydrated. It can be used as a meat substitute or as a filler in dishes such as meatloaf.

- tempeh, made from whole cooked soybeans formed into a chewy cake, and used as a meat substitute.

- miso, fermented soybean paste used for seasoning and in soup stock

- roasted soybean nuts made from whole roasted soybeans and used principally as a low calorie, high protein snack.

Other processed soy products sold widely in mainstream US grocery stores include:

- soy based burgers, meatballs, hotdogs and sausages

- soy cheese and cold cuts

- soy protein fortified pastas and cereals

Owing to the fact that soy products have a mild, or even a neutral or plain taste, they easily are incorporated into a "5 to 9 a day" plan by:

- thickening sauces and gravies with soy products

- adding soymilk to baked goods and desserts

- using tofu in stews, soups, and eaten in stir frys for lunch or dinners

- consuming soy based beverages, muffins, sausages, or yogurt for breakfast

- substituting soy deli cold cuts, soy nut butter, or soy cheese to make sandwiches using whole grain bread

- topping pizzas with soy cheese, sausages, or crumbles

- grilling soy dogs, burgers, or adding marinated tempeh or baked tofu to the menu

- cubing or stir frying tofu or tempeh to be added to a salad

- pouring soy milk on cereal, using it in cooking, or to make smoothies

- ordering soy based dishes such as bean curd and miso soups at Asian restaurants

- eating roasted soy nuts or a soy protein bar for a snack

The FDA has reviewed a number of studies that have demonstrated the value of a soy based diet and have approved a unique "soy health claim". Theses studies demonstrate the value of a diet based on soy protein in terms of lowering levels of total blood cholesterol and low density lipoprotein cholesterol. As a result, the FDA has determined that foods made with the whole soybean may qualify for the "soy health claim" if they have no fat other than that naturally present in the whole soy bean. This claim is basically as follows:

"Diets low in saturated fat and cholesterol that include 25 grams of soy protein a day may reduce the risk of heart disease. One serving (citing the name of the food) provides (specific number) grams of soy protein".

To qualify for this "soy health claim" foods must meet the following additional criteria per serving:

- 6.25 grams soy protein

- < 3 grams fat

- <1 gram saturated fat

- <20 milligrams cholesterol

- <480 milligrams sodium for individual foods, and

- <960 milligrams sodium if considered a meal

Scientific data strongly supports the nutritional value and health benefits of increasing soy protein in the diet. As the number of soy based products grows, it will become increasingly easy for individuals to add enough soy protein to their daily diets to meet the 25 gram amount that the FDA and the scientific literature indicates is beneficial to health. Examples of such existing products and their soy protein content are as follows:

Product	Soy Protein Content
• 4 ounces of firm tofu	13 grams
• one soy sausage link	6 grams
• one soy burger	10 grams
• 8 ounce glass soymilk	10 grams
• 1 soy protein bar	14 grams
• one half cup tempeh	19 grams
• ¼ cup roasted soy nuts	19 grams

Soybean products also are being promoted for their potential protective properties against breast, colon, endometrial, lung and prostate cancer. Anticancer effects of the soybean may be due to the isoflavone phytonutrients, genistein, and daidzein, found in soybeans and their products. Studies are being done to clarify the role of these phytonutrients in such cancers.

Additional soy information, history, health benefits/risks, research, adding soy to the diet, the soy health claim and more are available at: http://www.fda.gov/fdac/features/2000/300_soy.html

4.4.21 Mangos

The mango fruit is reported to have originated in Southeast Asia/India some 4000 years ago. Over time, mango groves spread to many tropical and subtropical parts of the world. Mango trees are evergreens growing up to 60 feet tall and fruiting 4 to 6 years after planting. They require hot, dry, periods to produce a good crop. There are more than 1,000 different varieties of mangos consumed throughout the world, and they come in different shapes, sizes, and coloring depending on ripeness. Colors range from yellow to green to orange or red, and they may weigh as little as a few ounces to a few pounds. They all have a rich tropical flavor when ripe. Most of the mangos sold in the United States today are imported from Mexico, Haiti, the Caribbean, and South America. Mangos offer the highest amount of beta carotene of any fruit. Beta carotene, a provitamin A antioxidant, is being studied chiefly for its potential role in the prevention of cancer and cardiovascular disease as well as other chronic disorders.

Serving is 1/2 a medium-sized mango (104 grams). A serving contains 70 calories, 0.5 gram fat and no cholesterol, sodium, calcium, iron, or protein. However, it has 17 grams of carbohydrate, 1 gram fiber, 15 grams sugars and 40% DV of vitamin A and 15% DV of vitamin C. The mango is considered to be a good source of vitamin A, and to a lesser extent, vitamin C.

Mangos are readily incorporated into a "5 to 9 a day" plan. Cut up a mango into chunks and add to any fruit salad or yogurt. Use mangos to top bagels with fat free cream cheese. Include mangos in a fruit shake or smoothie for a tropical treat.

Additional mango information, varieties, selection, preparation, inclusion in a "5 to 9 a day" plan and recipes are available at:
http://www.cdc.gov/nccdphp/dnpa/5aday/month/mango.htm

4.4.22 Mushrooms

Mushrooms are not a true vegetable in the sense that they do not have any leaves, roots or seeds and do not need any light to grow. Rather mushrooms are fungi that create more mushrooms by releasing spores. They are found all over the world, and ancient Egyptians considered them to be food for the royals. Thousands of mushroom varieties exist today. Some are edible and others are highly toxic. Agaricus (white or button) mushrooms are the most common variety prepackaged in supermarkets, and available fresh, canned or frozen. Portobello mushrooms, sometimes the size of a hamburger, are circular and flat with a dense chewy texture. They are sold fresh and are excellent for grilling or roasting.

Serving size is 5 medium mushrooms (84 grams). A serving contains 20 calories, and no fat, cholesterol, sodium, or sugars, 3 grams of protein, 3 grams of carbohydrate, and 1 gram of dietary fiber. Mushrooms are brimming with protein, B vitamins (riboflavin, niacin, and pantothenic acid), and minerals (selenium, potassium and copper). They are very low in calories, and may contain antibacterial phytonutrients that help the body ward off infections.

Mushrooms easily can be incorporated into a "5 to 9 a day" plan. Add sliced mushrooms to a salad, soup or pasta. They make an attractive addition to vegetable platters. Grill a portabello mushroom and have a healthy "veggie burger", adding lettuce and tomato to a whole wheat bun. Include mushrooms to stir frys. Make a homemade white pizza combo with low fat mozzarella topped with different kinds of mushrooms. Try mushrooms on a skewer with bell peppers, squash and pineapple.

It is best to buy mushrooms from a reputable grower or grocer instead of hunting them "in the wild", as there are many wild poisonous varieties. Poisonous mushrooms can lead to sweating, cramps, diarrhea, confusion, convulsions, liver damage or even death.

Additional mushroom information, varieties, selection, preparation, inclusion in a "5 to 9 a day" plan, and recipes area available at:
http://www.cdc.gov/nccdphp/dnpa/5aday/month/mushroom.htm

4.4.23 Onions

Onions are believed to have originated in Asia. Since early times, onions were one of the few vegetables that were recognized not to spoil during the winter months. The Egyptians worshiped the onion, believing that its spherical shape and concentric rings symbolized eternity. Today, onions are used in a variety of dishes and rank sixth among the world's leading vegetable crops. Onions come in three basic colors, yellow, red and white. Approximately 80-90% of the US onion crop is devoted to the yellow onion, and the other 10% or so to the red and white varieties.

Onions are low in calories and in most nutrients. However, they not only provide flavor in cooking, but also are a source of health promoting phytochemicals such as quercetin and alluim, both considered to be helpful in preventing cardiovascular disease and cancer.

Eating at least half an onion a day is reported to reduce the risk of stomach cancer by 50%. Scientists believe that this reduction is due at least in part, to sulfur containing compounds in onions that attack Helicobacter pylori, an infectious agent believed to be a causative factor for stomach cancers.

Serving size is 1 medium onion (148 grams). A serving contains 60 calories and has no fat, cholesterol or sodium. Total carbohydrate content is 14 grams (5% DV), dietary fiber 3 grams (12% DV), vitamin C (20% DV), calcium (4% DV) and iron (2% DV).

Onions are easily incorporated into a "5 to 9 a day" plan. Raw or cooked onions may be used to season stews, soups, tomato sauces, or cooked vegetables. Small pearl onions make a good side dish when seasoned with thyme. Baked or stuffed onions may be enjoyed on their own or as a snack. They may be stuffed with chopped vegetables, rice or bread crumbs. Raw onions may be added to salads or fresh vegetable trays, or added to provide crunch and flavor to dressings.

Additional onion information, history, selection, storage, varieties, preparation, inclusion in a "5 to 9 a day" plan and recipes are available at: http://www.cdc.gov/nccdphp/dnpa/5aday/month/onion.htm

4.4.24 Oranges

Orange trees are semitropical evergreens, seldom exceeding 30 feet in height, originating in Southeast Asia. By 1820, there were orange grooves in St Augustine, Florida. Today Florida is the number one citrus grower, producing 70% of the US orange crop, with 90% going into juice. Varieties include the sweet orange, sour orange, and mandarin orange or tangerine. The US produces the sweet variety, and Spain the sour, used in marmalades and liqueurs. The Navel orange is a seedless orange, with a medium thick rind, in which a second small, orange grows. That second small orange is technically a hesperidum, a kind of berry.

Serving size is 1 medium orange (154 grams/5.5 ounces). A serving contains 70 calories and no fat, cholesterol or sodium. Potassium content is 269 milligrams (7% DV), carbohydrate 21 grams (7% DV), dietary fiber 7 grams (28% DV), sugars 14 grams, protein 1 gram, vitamin C (130% DV), calcium (6% DV) and iron (2% DV).

Most of the consumption of oranges is in the form of juice. Eating the whole fruit provides 130% of the RDA for vitamin C, less than the juice, but more fiber, which is generally not present in the juice. The whole orange also is considered to be a good source of fiber and potassium.

Oranges may be made part of a "5 to 9 a day" plan in a variety of ways. Drink a cool glass of orange juice for breakfast or serve orange wedges instead of grapefruit for a change. Combine orange juice with other fruits and yogurt for a smoothie. Cut oranges into wedges and eat them for a light snack or as garnishes. Buy a zesting tool or grate orange rind to use in recipes, rice or stir fry for added flavor. Carry an orange with you and eat it as a snack. Orange juice can be used over fresh fruits to prevent "browning".

Additional orange information history, selection, storage, varieties, inclusion in a "5 to 9 a day" plan, and recipes are available at: http://www.cdc.gov/nccdphp/dnpa/5aday/month/orange.htm

4.4.25 Papayas

Papayas are believed to be native to Mexico and Central America. They are a melon like fruit with a yellow/orange flesh enclosed in a thin skin that varies in color from green to orange to rose. Today, papayas can be found all year long with the peak season being early summer and fall. Most papayas are imported from Hawaii, Central and South America. Two main types of papayas exist, the Hawaiian and Mexican. The Hawaiian varieties are known as Solo papayas. They are pear shaped, about 1 pound each, and have a yellow skin and an orange or pinkish flesh, when ripe. The Mexican varieties are not as common but can be found in Latino supermarkets. They are much large in size. This fruit contains an enzyme called papain, which may be used as a meat tenderizer.

Serving size is ½ small papaya (140 grams). A serving contains 70 calories and no fat, cholesterol, or protein. Carbohydrate content is 19 grams (6%), fiber 2 grams (10% DV), vitamin A (8% DV), vitamin C (150% DV), sugars 9 grams. Sodium, calcium, and iron content are low. One half of a small papaya can be a rich source of vitamin C and a good source of vitamin A as well as folate, fiber and potassium.

Papayas can be incorporated in a "5 to 9 a day" plan in a variety of ways. Use papayas to make a hot and spicy salsa. Blend papayas with milk, yogurt, or orange juice for a breakfast smoothie. Puree papayas to make a delicious salad dressing or base for a sorbet. Add papaya slices to honeydew, melon, and strawberries to make a colorful fruit cup or salad.

Additional information on papayas, varieties, selection, storage, inclusion in a "5 to 9 a day" plan and recipes are available at: http://www.cdc.gov/nccdphp/dnpa/5aday/month/papaya.htm

4.4.26 Passion Fruits

Native to Brazil, passion fruits consumed in the US are grown chiefly in Hawaii, California, and Florida. These sources, along with imports from New Zealand keep passion fruit on the market all year. They are an egg shaped tropical fruit that is also called a purple granadilla (means "little pomegranate" in Spanish). The seeds are edible and the orange pulp can be eaten straight from the shell. However, passion fruits are more commonly sieved and the highly aromatic pulp and juice are used as a flavoring for beverages and sauces. A number of varieties of passion fruit exist in 2 basic forms. New Zealand passion fruit is purple while the Hawaiian variety is yellow.

Serving size is 8 passion fruits (approximately ½ cup). A serving contains 140 calories, 1 gram total fat, 40 milligrams of sodium, 34 grams (11% DV) of total carbohydrate, 15 grams of dietary fiber (60% DV), 19 grams of sugars, 3 grams of protein, vitamin A (20% DV), vitamin C (70% DV), iron (12% DV), and calcium (2% DV). Passion fruits are regarded as a good source of vitamin

A and C, as well as potassium and iron. One passion fruit has only 16 calories. When eaten with the seeds, a serving is an excellent source of fiber.

Passion fruits may be made part of a "5 to 9 a day" plan by spooning this fruit over low fat yogurt to make a colorful treat, adding it to mixed green salads or fruit salads for a new taste, and topping chicken, fish or pork with a spoonful of passion fruit.

Additional passion fruit information, varieties, selection, preparation, inclusion in a "5 to 9 a day" plan and recipes are available at: http://www.cdc.gov/nccdphp/dnpa/5aday/month/passionfruit.htm

4.4.27 Peaches

Peaches, members of the rose family, were first cultivated in China in ancient times, and revered as a symbol of longevity. Travelers along caravan routes carried the peach seed to Europe. In the early 1700s, Spanish missionaries established peaches in California. Today, around half of the peach crop in the United States comes from the South, and the other half from California. The US produces around 25% of the total world market. Off season, peaches are imported into the US from Chile and Mexico. In the US, the season dictates the variety. Semi freestones (Queencrest) are early season, late April to June. By mid June, the market shifts to freestone (Elegant Lady) or clingstone. Fresh varieties are sold as freestone while clingstones are usually used for canning. The fruit inside these peaches is either yellow or white. The white flesh variety has a more sugary sweet flavor. The more traditional yellow variety is more acid and more flavorful.

Serving size is one medium peach (98 grams). A serving contains 40 calories and no fat, cholesterol, iron, calcium, or sodium. Carbohydrate content is 10 grams (3% DV), dietary fiber 2 grams (8% DV), sugars 9 grams, protein 1 gram, vitamin A (2% DV), and vitamin C (10% DV). Whether fresh, canned or frozen, peaches are nutritious, being fat, cholesterol and sodium free with significant amounts of vitamin C.

Peaches may be incorporated into a "5 to 9 a day" plan in a variety of ways. Add sliced peaches to cereal, or as a topper to pancakes or waffles. Take a peach or a cup of canned peaches to work for a healthy snack. Include peaches in low fat yogurt or cottage cheese and put on toast. Combine peaches and other fresh fruits into a fruit salad. Make a peach smoothie with yogurt and peaches in a blender for breakfast or a snack. Bake, grill or broil peaches and serve along with meat or fish dinners. Freeze a can of peaches in the freezer, then open and blend in a blender for a great summer dessert sorbet.

Additional peach information, varieties, selection, storage, use, inclusion in a "5 to 9 a day" plan, and recipes are available at: http://www.cdc.gov/nccdphp/dnpa/5aday/month/peach.htm

4.4.28 Pears

Pears (Pyrus communis) are a pome fruit and relative of the apple. Homer referred to pears as "Gifts from the Gods". Pears arrived in the US in the 1700s and now rank second to the apple as the most popular fruit. They can be eaten or used as a food in much the same ways as the apple. There are now 3000 or so known varieties in the world. US production comes from the Northwest, New York, Pennsylvania, Michigan, and California. Imports come from South America, Canada, New Zealand, and South Africa. With numerous varieties, extended growing seasons, and imports, pears of all sizes and colors are available all year. Varieties of pears include the Anjou, Bartlett, Bose, Comice, Forelle and Seckel. They have a sweet, rich flavor and come in a variety of colors including green, golden yellow and red.

Serving size is one medium sized pear. Pears have no cholesterol, sodium, or saturated fat. They offer a natural quick source of energy largely due to two monosacharides, glucose and fructose, the sweetest of known natural sugars. Carbohydrates make up to 98% of the energy provided by a pear. A fresh pear serving offers 6 grams of fiber, much of it in the form of pectin, 210 milligrams of potassium and 7 milligrams of vitamin C (10% of the RDA). Pears are considered to be good source of fiber, potassium and vitamin C.

Pears can readily be incorporated into a "5 to 9 a day" plan. They make a good snack. Baked or broiled pears can be used with a sauce as a light, tasty dessert. Pear slices dipped in lemon can be used as a garnish. Thin sliced wedges can be served with chunks of cheese, turkey and grapes on a skewer to make a healthy appetizer or side dish. Toss chopped pears into a chicken, tuna, greens, fruit or cottage cheese salads. Try pear slices in a grilled chicken sandwich. Substitute pears for apples in recipes.

Additional pear information, varieties, selection, storage, incorporation into a "5 to 9 a day" plan, and recipes are available at: http://www.cdc.gov/nccdphp/dnpa/5aday/month/pear.htm

4.4.29 Peas/Fresh

Green peas are members of the legume family that includes plants that bear pods enclosing fleshy seeds. They do not need the long cooking times that are required by dried legumes such as split peas and beans. While dried peas have been in use since ancient times, it was not until the sixteenth century that more tender green pea varieties were developed and eaten fresh. Today only about 5% of all peas grown are sold fresh. More than half of all peas sold are canned and the rest are frozen. Fresh green peas need to be refrigerated or half their sugar content may turn to starch within six hours.

Serving size is ½ cup of fresh peas (frozen, cooked). A serving contains 63 calories and has no cholesterol or sodium. Carbohydrate content is 12 grams, dietary fiber 4 grams (14% DV), protein 4 grams, total fat 0.2 gram, vitamin A (10% DV), vitamin C (13% DV), iron (14% DV), thiamine (16% DV), folate (12% DV), and calcium (2% DV). Peas are regarded as a good low calorie source of non meat protein. A 100 calorie serving of peas (about ¾ cup) contains more protein than a whole egg or a tablespoon of peanut butter and has less than one gram of fat and no cholesterol.

Snow peas (Chinese pea pods) and sugar snap peas can be eaten raw as a snack or cooked with the pod intact. Snow peas supply less protein and are lower in B vitamins than green shelled peas because they are eaten when their seeds are still immature. However, snow peas provide almost twice the calcium, 100% of the RDA for vitamin C, and slightly more iron than green peas.

Peas can be incorporated into a "5 to 9 a day" plan in a variety of ways such as:

- season cooked peas with fresh or dried mint, chopped fresh parsley or with lemon

- add shelled green peas, snow or sugar snap peas to tossed green salads or stir fried dishes

- eat snow or sugar snap peas raw or with a favorite low fat dip

- in a vegetable soup.

Additional fresh pea information, varieties, selection, storage, preparation, inclusion in a "5 to 9 a day" plan, and recipes are available at: http://www.cdc.gov/nccdphp/dnpa/5aday/month/peas.html

4.4.30 Peppers/Bell

Bell peppers can be found in a rainbow of colors and can vary in flavor. The variety of the pepper plant and the stage of ripeness determine the color and flavor of each pepper. A red pepper is simply a mature green bell pepper. As a bell pepper ages, its flavor becomes sweeter and milder. Red bell peppers have three times as much vitamin C and eleven times more beta carotene compared with the green varieties.

Serving size is ½ cup of green bell pepper (75 grams/2.7 ounces). A serving of green contains 20 calories, 0.14 gram total fat and no saturated fat or cholesterol. Carbohydrate content is 5 grams, dietary fiber 1.4 grams, sugars 2 grams, protein 1 gram, vitamin A 5% DV and vitamin C 12% DV. In contrast, a serving of red bell pepper contains 47% DV vitamin A, and 236% DV vitamin C. Thus, bell peppers are regarded as an excellent source of vitamin C and beta carotene, which play important roles in preventing some cancers, cardiovascular disease and other chronic disorders.

Bell peppers are easily incorporated into a "5 to 9 a day" plan. Mix different colored, sliced, or chopped peppers into salads, pastas, and Chinese and Mexican dishes, or add then as colorful garnishes. Include sliced peppers on a vegetable tray. Stuff peppers with whole grain brown rice or use them as colorful containers for dips or other edible items.

Additional bell pepper information, varieties, selection, storage, inclusion in a "5 to 9 a day" plan, and recipes are available at: http://www.cdc.gov/nccdphp/dnpa/5aday/month/bell_pepper.htm

4.4.31 Pineapples

The word pineapple is derived from *pina*, the Spanish word used to describe a pinecone. They were introduced to the Hawaiian Islands, now the leading producers of this fruit. There are four types of pineapples. These include the Gold, Smooth Cayenne, Red Spanish, and Sugar Loaf. They are sold fresh and canned and all have a sweet flavor. The Gold variety has an extra sweet flavor, golden color, and higher vitamin C content.

Serving size is 2 slices of pineapple (112 grams/4 ounces). A serving contains 60 calories, no fat or cholesterol, 10 milligrams sodium, 115 milligrams potassium (3% DV), 16 grams carbohydrate (5% DV), 1 gram dietary fiber (4% DV), 1 gram protein, and 13 grams sugars, 25% DV of vitamin C and 2% DV of both calcium and iron.

Pineapples are easy to include in a "5 to 9 a day" plan. Drink a glass of pineapple juice for breakfast. Eat a slice of pineapple topped with cottage cheese or add some to your low fat pizza.

Additional pineapple information, varieties, selection, storing, inclusion in a "5 to 9 a day" plan, and recipes are available at:
http://www.cdc.gov/nccdphp/dnpa/5aday/month/pineapple.htm

4.4.32 Plums/Prunes

The word plum is derived from the Latin prunum meaning a plum. Plums are native to China, Europe and America. The Romans apparently introduced this fruit into Northern Europe. There are more than 200 varieties of plums that vary in size, color, and taste. European, Japanese (formerly Chinese), Damsons, and Mirabelles, and "cherry plums" are the main varieties of plums. Plum trees grow up to 15-21 feet high, have greenish-white flowers, are pollinated by bees, and drop their leaves in autumn. Plums are somewhat high in carbohydrates and low in fat., protein, sodium and calories. A serving is considered to be a fairly good source of vitamin A, potassium and phytonutrients.

Plums contain a substance in their skin that produces a laxative action. If the plum is peeled, this laxative effect can largely be avoided, if desired. Prunes, dried plums, also contain this chemical substance, hydroxyphenylisatin, that works as a gentle stimulant laxative. Dietary fiber content of prunes also aids in this laxative effect. Prune juice also is a reasonably effective laxative without the dietary fiber content. Prunes and prune juice are time honored home remedies for constipation.

A serving is approximately five prunes (¼ cup, 40 grams). It contains around 110 calories, no fat or cholesterol, 5 milligrams sodium, 290 milligrams potassium (8% DV), 26 grams carbohydrate (11% DV), 2 grams dietary fiber (9% DV), 13 grams sugars, 1 gram protein, 10% DV vitamin A, 4% DV vitamin C and 4% DV iron.

Both plums and prunes contain antioxidants that help neutralize the damaging effects of free radicals, and play a role in the prevention of the aging process, development of certain cancers, as well as cardiovascular disease, lung disorders, and cataract formation.

The USDA Human Nutrition Research Center at Tufts University tested and ranked the antioxidant activity of commonly eaten fruits and vegetables using the ORAC method (Oxygen Radical Absorbency Capacity). Prunes topped the list in ORAC scores, having more than twice the antioxidant capacity as other high scoring fruits such as blueberries and raisins. In fact, the antioxidant activity of prunes was found to be approximately 6 times greater than plums and around twice that of blueberries and raisins, next on the list. ORAC values found were reported to be as follows:

Fruits	ORAC Value	Vegetables	ORAC Value
prunes	5770	kale	1770
raisins	2830	spinach	1260
blueberries	2400	brussels sprouts	980
blackberries	2036	broccoli flowers	890
strawberries	1540	beets	840
raspberries	1220		
plums	949		

oranges	750
pink grapefruit	483
cantaloupe	252
apples	218
pears	134

http://www.sunsweet.com/nutrition.cfm
http://www.californiadriedplums.org/consumer/nutrition_aoxscores.asp

Neochologenic acid is a potent phenolic antioxidant of the hydroxycinnamate family found in significant amounts in fresh plums and prunes. Half the amount of this compound survives the drying and processing required to convert plums into prunes. A serving of prunes is reported to provide around 70 milligrams of total phenolic compounds, mostly hydroxycinnamic acids, that serve as free radical scavengers diminishing cellular damage that may lead to cancer, cardiovascular disease, cataracts, and other age related chronic disorders. For additional information, see:
http://www.californiadriedplums.org/consumer/nutrition_phenolic.asp

The glycemic index of a food describes its relative ability to influence blood sugar levels compared to white bread, with its baseline score set at 100. Although prunes contain some sugars (fructose, glucose, and sorbitol), they are reported to have almost no sucrose. In addition, dietary fiber in prunes may help modulate the body's uptake of sugar from prunes. These factors may help explain the favorably low glycemic index of 54 for prunes compared to 100 for white bread. Thus, prunes may be regarded as an appropriate fruit for inclusion in a diabetic diet. For additional information see:
http://www.californiadriedplums.org/consumer/nutrition_glycemic.asp

For individuals with high blood pressure or other medical conditions that may benefit from increased potassium intake, prunes/prune juice may be appropriate. The FDA now allows certain potassium rich foods to make a health claim that states on the nutrition label:
"Diets containing foods that are good sources of potassium and low in sodium may reduce the risk of high blood pressure and stroke."

To quality for this potassium health claim, a food must:

- have at least 350 milligrams of potassium per "reference amount customarily consumed (RACC)". For prune juice, RACC is 8 ounces or 240 milliliters.

- have 140 milligrams or less of sodium

- be low in fat, saturated fat and cholesterol

Eight ounces of prune juice provides 540 milligrams or 15% of the Daily Value (3500 milligrams) for potassium and meets the other requirements. Thus, prune juice qualifies for this health claim. Prunes, on the other hand, do not quite measure up to these requirements for this health claim, but still are regarded as a good food source for potassium.

Prunes are easily incorporated into a "5 to 9 a day" plan. They are a versatile ingredient in appetizers, salads, desserts, and stir fries.

Additional information on prunes is available at:
http://www.californiadriedplums.org
http://www.5aday.com/html/educators/insights_holder.php?columns=plums1

4.4.33 Squash

Squash is reported to have been a dietary staple for Native Americans and was a mainstay food for early Europeans who settled in America. George Washington and Thomas Jefferson were reported to be enthusiastic squash growers. Many new varieties have been added from other parts of the world, and this has resulted in the variety of colors, shapes, and sizes that are available today. Some varieties of squash grow on vines while others grow on bushes. Squash are commonly divided into two groups, summer and winter. Several types of summer squash exist, but zucchini is the most popular in the US. Squash are fleshy vegetables protected by a hard rind. They belong to the plant family that includes melons and cucumbers. Coumarins and flavonoids are the chief types of phytonutrients found in squash. The skin and rind of summer squash are rich in the nutrient beta carotene whereas the fleshy portion of this vegetable is not. To gain the full nutritional benefits of squash, the skins and rinds should be eaten.

Serving size is ½ medium squash (98 grams). A serving contains 20 calories and no fat, cholesterol or sodium. Total carbohydrate content is 4 grams, dietary fiber 2 grams, sugars 2 grams, protein 1 gram, vitamin A (6% DV), vitamin C (30% DV) and calcium and iron 2% DV.

Squash can be incorporated into a "5 to 9 a day" plan in a variety of ways:

- cook several varieties/colors of summer squash together to make a colorful side dish

- add favorite seasonings (dill, lemon juice, etc.) to summer squash that has been steamed, sautéed, or grilled

- include yellow and zucchini squash in a vegetable tray

- put sliced squash with tomatoes into rice when cooking it

- sliced or grated squash can be added to a salad

- grated summer squash makes a good substitute for carrots in a carrot cake

Additional squash information, varieties, selection, storage, incorporation in a "5 to 9 a day" plan, and recipes are available at:
http://www.cdc.gov/nccdphp/dnpa/5aday/month/squash.htm

4.4.34 Sweet Potatoes

Sweet potatoes are a Native American vegetable and were the main source of nourishment for early homesteaders and soldiers during the Revolutionary War. Their tuberous roots are regarded as among the more nutritious foods in the vegetable kingdom. Even though the sweet potato is not a yam, it is acceptable to use the term yam when referring to sweet potatoes. There are two main varieties of sweet potatoes, the pale yellow with a dry flesh, and the dark orange with a moist flesh. The dark orange variety is plumper in shape and somewhat sweeter than the yellow variety. They are considered to be good sources of potassium and vitamins A and C. Sweet potatoes also contain an enzyme that converts most of its starches into sugars as the potato matures, and this sweetness continues to increase during storage when they are cooked.

Serving size is 3.5 ounces of sweet potato (1.5 cups shredded). A serving contains 140 calories, no fat or cholesterol, 24 milligrams of sodium, 195 milligrams potassium, 6 grams carbohydrate, 2 grams dietary fiber, 3 grams sugars, 1 gram protein, 15% DV vitamin A, 47% DV vitamin C and small amounts of calcium and iron.

Sweet potatoes may easily be incorporated in a "5 to 9 a day" plan by:

- using them in soups, casseroles, puddings, baked goods, or as a substitute for white potatoes in various recipes

- adding them to stir fries by cutting them into thin sticks so that they cook quickly.

Additional sweet potato information, varieties, selection, preparation, storage, inclusion in a "5 to 9 a day" plan and recipes are available at: http://www.cdc.gov/nccdphp/dnpa/5aday/month/sweet_potato.htm

4.4.35 Tomatoes

Currently, tomatoes are regarded as one of the most popular vegetables in the United States. Tomatoes are members of the fruit family but they are served and prepared as a vegetable and this may be the reason why most people consider them to be a vegetable and not a fruit. There are literally thousands of varieties of tomato. The most widely available varieties in the US are classified in three groups: cherry, plum and slicing tomatoes. A new sweet variety, the grape tomato, is a very tasty variety to eat alone or in a salad.

Tomatoes are high in vitamin C and lycopene, both potent antioxidants. The National Cancer Institute published a study that showed an association between consuming a diet rich in tomato based foods and a decreased risk of prostate cancer which may be due to their lycopene content. Antioxidants such as lycopene have been reported to prevent cancer and cardiovascular as well as other chronic diseases. Tomato paste and sauces are rich in lycopene not only because they are more concentrated but also because cooking tomatoes "releases" tightly bound lycopene, facilitating absorption from the intestines.

Studies have shown that daily consumption of tomato products providing at least 40 milligrams of lycopene may be enough to substantially reduce low density lipoprotein (LDL) oxidation and damaging free radical production. High LDL oxidation is associated with increased risk of cardiovascular disease. Adequate lycopene levels can be achieved by drinking just two glasses of tomato juice a day. Other research suggests that lycopene can reduce the risk of prostate cancer and cancers of the lung, bladder, cervix, breast and skin. A review of 72 studies by Harvard Medical School, found that 57 of them linked tomato products intake with a reduced risk of cancers, and in 35 of these the association was strong enough to be considered statistically significant. Individuals who consumed at least 10 weekly servings of tomato based foods were up to 45% less likely to develop prostate cancer.

Serving size is 1 medium tomato (148 grams). A serving contains 35 calories, 0.5 gram total fat, no saturated fat or cholesterol, 5 milligrams sodium, 7 grams total carbohydrate, 1 gram dietary fiber, 4 grams sugars, 1 gram protein, 20% DV vitamin A, 40% DV vitamin C, 2% DV calcium and 2% DV iron.

Tomatoes easily can be incorporated into a "5 to 9 a day" plan in a variety of ways. They can be enjoyed fresh, stuffed, baked, stewed or grilled. Add one to a sandwich, salad, or omelet. Try broiled tomatoes topped with basil leaves. Tomatoes make an excellent base for homemade soups or sauces and especially compliment pasta dishes. Raw tomatoes can make a tasty Mexican salsa. Tomatoes combine well with just about any type of food such as poultry, fish, rice, pasta and other vegetables. Combine tomatoes with other vegetables to make a tasty side dish or snack.

Additional tomato information, varieties, storage, selection, preparation, inclusion in a "5 to 9 a day" plan, and recipes are available at:
http://www.cdc.gov/nccdphp/dnpa/5aday/month/tomato.htm
http://www.leffingwell.com/lycopene.htm
http://www.cornell.edu/cce.htm (search "tomatoes")

4.4.36 Watermelons

Watermelons can be traced back to Africa as part of the cucumber and squash family. Early watermelons were small and mainly rind and seeds. Today's varieties are larger, sweeter, and have smaller seeds, and a thinner rind. Watermelon is 92% water and 8% sugar, so it is aptly named, and remains among the most refreshing and thirst quenching fruits of all. There are more than 50 varieties of watermelon. Most have red flesh, but there are orange and yellow fleshed varieties. Of the 50 or so varieties of watermelon available in the US, there are four general categories: Allsweet, Ice Box, Seedless, and Yellow Flesh.

Nutritionists have long appreciated the health benefits watermelon provides, particularly as a good source of vitamins A and C, as well as fiber. Recently, research has shed new light on watermelon's health benefits due to high concentrations of lycopene, an antioxidant that may help reduce the risks of cancer, cardiovascular disease, and other chronic disorders. Further discussion of the health benefits of lycopene is available at: http://www.leffingwell.com/lycopene/htm

Serving size is 2 cups of diced watermelon, 1/18 medium melon (280 grams). A serving contains 80 calories, no fat or cholesterol, 10 milligrams sodium (<1% DV), 27 grams total carbohydrate (11% DV), 2 grams dietary fiber (8% DV), 25 grams sugars, 1 gram protein, 20% DV of vitamin A, 25% DV vitamin C, 2% DV calcium and 4% DV iron.

Watermelon easily can be incorporated into a "5 to 9 a day" plan by:

- keeping watermelon chunks, slices or juice in the refrigerator for snacks or as a thirst quencher

- combining it with other fruits an appetizer, or in fresh fruit salad or as a dessert

Additional watermelon information, varieties, selection, tips, storing, inclusion in a "5 to 9 a day" plan and recipes are available at: http://www.cdc.gov/nccdphp/dnpa/5aday/month/watermelon.htm

4.5 Seeds/Nuts

4.5.1. Introduction

Seeds and nuts are regarded as good sources of protein, carbohydrates, vitamins, minerals, disease preventive phytonutrients, and healthy unsaturated fat. They also add variety to "5 to 9 a day" eating plans by offering nutrition alternatives. Studies suggest that a handful of seeds or nuts a day is associated with a significant reduction in cardiovascular disease. Both seeds and nuts are high in calories so don't "go nuts" eating them. Rather, try and mix them with other foods in a balanced diet to help keep calories regulated satisfactorily and still allow for enjoyment and good nutrition.

Seeds are regarded as the initial and final turning points in the life of plants, generating new specimens/life. Fruits keep seeds carefully protected on the inside, arranged for taste. Aside from being rich in vitamins, minerals and phytonutrients, 100 grams of seeds contain around 650 calories and 25 to 30 grams of protein as well as a good source of the essential omega-3 fatty acids. Sesame and sunflower seeds also are excellent sources of calcium. Flaxseeds also are high in omega-3 essential unsaturated fatty acids, and in addition, they also act as an "intestinal tract regulator" owing to their high fiber content.

Cocoa, the seed of the cocoa tree, was considered sacred by the Mayans and Aztecs before the Europeans invented chocolate by adding refined sugar. However, cocoa powder still remains a basic ingredient in the American diet. Unsweetened and with a small fat content, cocoa intake still needs to be moderated because of its high calorie content.

Nuts are the kind of seed that fills the space inside the fruit. They are an excellent source for essential polyunsaturated fatty acids. Walnuts are reported to have the richest vitamin E content, about 3 milligrams per 100 grams of walnuts. Pistachio nuts have the highest protein content, around 20 grams per 100 grams of pistachios. The Brazil nut, the Queen of the chestnuts, has the highest selenium content. Chestnuts are among the lowest in fat content, having around 2 grams total fat per serving.

Research has consistently shown that individuals who routinely consume seeds and nuts have a significantly reduced rate of cardiovascular disease, attributed in part at least, to lower blood levels of cholesterol produced. Almonds and walnuts appear to be the most effective in this regard.

A number of nutritional factors in nuts may be responsible for this protection against cardiovascular disease offered by seeds and nuts. These may include, fiber, vitamin E, alpha linolenic acid (found primarily in walnuts), oleic acid, magnesium, potassium and arginine. However, exactly how nuts lower the risk of cardiovascular disease remains to be determined.

4.5.2 Walnuts

Walnuts are regarded as unique among nuts because their fat is polyunsaturated, and an important source of essential omega-3 fatty acids (that lower cholesterol and protect against cardiovascular disease). Individuals experience as much as a 12% drop in total cholesterol and a 16% decrease in low density lipoprotein (LDL) cholesterol when walnuts are substituted for some of the saturated fat in the diet,. Polyphenol rich extracts from walnuts also are reported to decrease in vitro plasma LDL oxidation and free radical formation. Walnuts substituted for some of the monounsaturated fat in the Mediterranean diet, are reported to produce even more lowering of blood cholesterol levels. Five to six walnuts a day may be sufficient for such beneficial effects.

Available evidence indicates that omega-3s lower cholesterol and protect against heart disease and some cancers, and help ease symptoms of arthritis. Omega-3 fatty acids are found in cold water fish such as salmon, flaxseed, leafy green vegetables, plant foods including walnuts, and soybeans. Omega-3s also prevent platelets from sticking together and blood from clotting, and some studies show that they not only decrease the risk of heart attacks but also stroke.

The omega-3 content of naturally occurring foods is reported to be as follows:

Fish sources	Amount*	Plant Food	Amount*
Mackerel, Atlantic	2.6 grams	Flaxseed	18.0

Trout, lake	2.0 grams	Walnuts, English	6.8
Herring, Atlantic	1.7 grams	Soybeans, raw	3.4
Sturgeon, Atlantic	1.5 grams	Soybeans, dry	1.6
Tuna, Albacore	1.5 grams	Oats, Germs	1.4
Salmon, Atlantic	1.5 grams	Spinach, raw	0.9
Bluefish	1.2 grams	Wheat, germ	0.7
Bass, stripped	0.8 gram	Purslane	0.4
Halibut, Pacific	0.5 grams	Kale, raw	0.3
		Broccoli, raw	0.2

*Amounts are in grams of omega-3 fatty acid per 100 grams of food source.

While a 4:1 or less ratio of omega-6 to omega-3 fatty acids appears to be best for optimal health, many supermarket products consumed by Americans contain from 14 to 20 times more omega-6 than omega-3 fatty acids upsetting a so called critical nutritional balance and incurring a greater risk for virtually all the diseases referred to as "the diseases of civilization." Fortunately, English walnuts have an ideal balance of omega-3 to omega-6 fatty acids.

Serving size is 5-7 walnuts or 10-14 walnut halves containing about 130-180 calories.

Walnuts are easily incorporated into a "5 to 9 a day" plan. They add appeal, taste, and crunch to a wide variety of dishes from snacks and appetizers to salads and entries. This versatility allows one to add a handful serving of walnuts (around 10 halves) to dietary intake every day as a snack or a side dish mixed with raisins.

Additional walnut information, history, health benefits, inclusion in a "5 to 9 a day" plan, and recipes are available at:
http://www.walnut.org/health/han_benefits.shtml

4.5.3 Peanuts

Peanuts are not nuts per se but a kind of bean. However, they are being considered here since they generally are regarded as nuts in America.

Peanuts contain significant amounts of omega-3, fatty acids, protein, fiber, vitamin E, folate, potassium, magnesium and zinc, all of which are regarded as important to health. They also contain phytonutrients such as phytosterols, flavonoids, and other antioxidants that also are regarded as beneficial to health. Like all plant foods, peanuts and peanut butter are cholesterol free.

A small handful of peanuts (1/2 ounce or about 17 peanuts) constitutes a serving of around 160 calories.

Peanuts and peanut butter servings are reported to:

- have undetectable levels of trans fats even though labels list partially hydrogenated oil as a minor ingredient

- contain about 7-8 grams of plant protein per serving and are rich in the amino acid arginine, which may aid in the prevention of cardiovascular disease by keeping blood vessels open through a vasodilating effect

- provide 2 grams of dietary fiber per one ounce serving. Peanut butter on a slice of whole grain bread provides about 4 grams of fiber.

- supply more eating satisfaction and feelings of fullness than carbohydrate snacks such as cookies, cake, crackers, chips or rice cakes.

Peanuts contain significant amounts of the phytonutrient, resveratrol, a polyphenol compound that is reported to reduce the risk of blood clots, cardiovascular disease, and cancer, etc. Red grapes also have resveratrol but it takes about 1.5 cups of grapes to equal the resveratrol in a ½ ounce packet of peanuts (about 17 peanuts).

Additional peanut information, research findings, health benefits, and use in a "5 to 9 a day" plan are available at:
http://www.peanut-institute.org
http://www.peanut-institute.org/HealthyDiets.html

4.5.4 Chestnuts

Chestnuts have been consumed for centuries in the Mediterranean area and Asia. Over 100 varieties of chestnut trees now exist, many of which produce clusters of small nuts (chatignes) whereas others produce single chestnuts, known in France as marrons. Chestnuts are related to the beechnut and the chinkapin, a nut eaten previously by Native Americans. Chestnuts are quite different from other nuts in that they are low in fat and contain a high starch content. They have a crumbly texture, and a sweet mild flavor. The horse chestnut is an inedible variety and not included in this discussion.

Serving size is 5 chestnuts containing around 103 calories. Chestnuts are composed of 6% water, 11% protein, 74% carbohydrate, 7% fat and 2.2% minerals. A serving contains 206 calories, 2.7 grams of protein, 44 grams carbohydrate, 1.8 grams total fat, 4.3 grams of fiber, vitamin B-6 (0.4 milligrams), vitamin C (22 milligrams), potassium (50 milligrams) and folate (59 milligrams). Chestnuts provide 8% of their calories as fat compared to macadamias with 95% as fat, pecans 91%, walnuts 87%, almonds 80% and peanuts 76%.

Chestnuts are easily incorporated into a "5 to 9 a day" plan. They are usually eaten boiled or roasted, and often added to soups or stuffings, or served as a side dish. They may be used to make a meringue dessert. Peeled whole chestnuts are available canned in water. They can be ground into flower and used for baking.

Additional chestnut information, history, varieties, buying and storing, preparation, tips, nutritional highlights, health benefits, inclusion in a "5 to 9 a day" plan and recipes are available at:
http://www.vitamin-galore.com/Food_Guide/Chestnuts.htm
http://www.dailybread.co.uk/food/chestnut.htm
http://www.chestnutfarms.com/cgi/peeled_frozen_chestnuts

A report entitled *The Effects of Fish Oils and Nuts on Health* by Claffey, Kocak and Rank is available at:
http://www.wfu.edu/users/clafmeO/fish%20oils.ppt

5. Dietary Supplements

5.1 Introduction

The term dietary supplement is defined by the United States Congress in the Dietary Supplement Health and Education Act (DSHEA) of 1994 as a product taken by mouth that contains an ingredient intended to supplement an individual's diet. Ingredients may include such things as vitamins, minerals, phytonutrients, herbs, or other substances taken as capsules, gelcaps, liquids, concentrates, tablets, powders, or other forms such as a food snack bar. DSHEA places dietary supplements in a special category under the umbrella of "foods", and requires that each be labeled as a "dietary supplement". A summary of DSHEA is available from the FDA at:
http://www.cfsan.fda.gov/~dms/dietsupp.html

Generally, manufacturers do not need to register with the FDA or obtain FDA approval before producing or selling dietary supplements. Thus, FDA regulation is "much looser" with dietary supplements compared with prescription or over the counter drugs.

An "Overview of Dietary Supplements" is provided by the FDA Center for Food Safety and Applied Nutrition, at:
http://www.cfsan.fda.gov/~dms/ds-oview.html

5.2 Classification of Ingredients

Ingredients in a dietary supplement are classified under DSHEA as either "established" or "new". In order for an ingredient to be "established", it must be one, or any combination of substances sold as a dietary supplement prior to October 15, 1994. A "new" dietary ingredient would be one that was not sold before October 15, 1994.

5.3 FDA Regulation/Labeling

The Federal Food, Drug and Cosmetic Act was amended by DSHEA creating a new framework for regulation of the safety and labeling of dietary supplements. Manufacturers or distributors now are responsible for determining that a dietary supplement is safe and that any representations or claims are substantiated by adequate evidence that such is not false or misleading. Dietary supplements containing established ingredients marketed before October 15, 1994 do not need FDA approval before they are marketed whereas those containing a new dietary ingredient, require premarket review for safety, claims, and other information required by law.

The FDA intends, from time to time, to issue new regulations regarding good manufacturing practices that ensure the identity, purity, quality, strength, and composition of dietary supplements in the future.

No authoritative complete list of "established" dietary ingredients that were marketed prior to October 15, 1994 exists at this time.

Manufacturers and distributors remain responsible for determining whether a dietary ingredient is new or not. Also, the manufacturer is responsible for establishing its own guidelines to insure that the dietary supplement it produces is safe and contains the ingredient(s) listed on the label.

Information required to appear on dietary supplement labels includes: descriptive name of the product, stating that it is a "supplement", plus the name and place of business of the manufacturer or distributor, a complete list of ingredients and the net contents of the product. The label must clearly identify each dietary ingredient contained in the product. Those ingredients not listed on the "supplemental facts" panel must be listed under "other ingredients" beneath the panel. Types of ingredients listed may include the source of the dietary ingredient (e.g., rose hips as the source of vitamin C), other food ingredients (e.g., water and sugar), and technical additives or processing aids (e.g. gelatin, starch, coloring agents, etc.). Other than the manufacturer's responsibility to ensure safety, there are no rules that limit serving size or the amount of an ingredient in a dietary supplement. Serving size is a decision determined by the manufacturer or distributor, and does not require FDA review or approval. For more detailed information than the label provides, the manufacturer or distributor needs to be contacted directly.

Unlike drug products, manufacturers and distributors of dietary supplements are not required by law to record, investigate, or forward to the FDA any reports they receive of injuries or illnesses that may be related to the use of their products. Once a dietary supplement is marketed, the FDA has the burden/responsibility to show that any given dietary supplement is "unsafe" before it can take action to restrict the product's use or remove it from the market, usually a difficult and long drawn out process at best. Also, there is no provision under any law or regulation enforced by the FDA that requires a manufacturer or distributor to disclose to the FDA or consumers the information they have about the safety or purported benefits of their dietary supplement product(s).

5.4 Tips/Dietary Supplement Users

Consumers and healthcare providers need to be well informed about dietary supplements before using them. Since it often is difficult to know what information is reliable, one may first want to contact the manufacturer, their healthcare provider and then the Web for appropriate information.

The FDA provides the following Websites for this purpose, namely:

* Guide to Dietary Supplements

  http://www.cfsan.fda.gov/~dms/fdsupp.html

* Dietary Supplements: Overview

  http://www.cfsan.fda.gov/~dms/supplmnt.html

5.5 Dietary Supplement Claims

The FDA's Center for Food Safety and Applied Nutrition (CFSAN) is responsible for this agency's oversight and regulation of dietary supplements, however limited it may be presently. Owing to limited resources, first priorities include mostly public health emergencies and products that may already have caused injury and illness. Next, products believed to be potentially unsafe or, illegal for any reason, receive the FDA's attention and enforcement efforts. Remaining funds/time are directed towards recalls, etc. The FDA does not analyze dietary supplements for content, etc. either before they are sold or in response to a consumer request.

No product sold as a dietary supplement may be promoted on its label as a treatment, prevention, or cure for any specific disease or condition. In this regard, it is important to bear in mind that labeling claims refers not only to the product label itself, but also to any accompanying material that is used by a manufacturer or distributor to promote and market the product.

The responsibility for ensuring the validity of any claims made for a dietary supplement rests with the manufacturer/distributor and the FDA. In case of advertising, such responsibility rests with the Federal Trade Commission (FTC).

By law, only three types of claims can be made for a dietary supplement. These are:

- health

- structure/function

- nutrient content

Claims made may describe the:

- link between a food substance and a disease or health related condition

- intended health benefits in using the product

- amount of a nutrient or dietary substance in the product.

When a manufacturer or distributor makes a structure/function claim (describing the role of a nutrient or dietary ingredient intended to affect the structure or function of the body) on a dietary supplement label, the applicable label must state that "this statement has not been evaluated by the FDA", and "the product is not intended to diagnose, treat, cure, or prevent any disease".

5.6 Advertisement Regulation

The FTC (Federal Trade Commission) regulates advertising including informericals, for dietary supplements, and the FDA works closely with the FTC in this area. However, the FTC's work is governed by different laws. Advertising and promotional material received in the mail also are regulated under different laws and are subject to regulation by the US Postal Service. Additional information in this regard is available at:
http://www.ftc.gov/bcp/menu-health.htm

5.7 Adverse Events Reporting

Any serious adverse event or illness attributable to any dietary supplement should be reported online to the nearest FDA District Office consumer complaint coordinator at:
http://www.fda.gov/medwatch/report/hcp.htm

5.8 Recent Information on Dietary Supplements

Recent information on Dietary Supplements is available at:
http://www.cfsan.fda.gov/~dms/supplmnt.html

5.9 Center for Food Safety and Applied Nutrition

CFSAN's Office of Nutritional Products, Labeling and Dietary Supplements (ONPLDS), recently was realigned. This Office is now organized by product categories to better align and coordinate staff activities, and features a separate unit for Dietary Supplements.

A report entitled: "Economic Characterization of the Dietary Supplement Industry" is available at:
http://vm.cfsan.fda.gov/~comm/ds-econ4.html

In this report, health benefits and toxicity of dietary supplement products involving various uses are discussed. Dietary supplements based on essential vitamins and minerals and their use in deficiency states are reviewed.

A partial list of popular herbal products made from leaves and stems of plants as well as other botanical products made from any other part of the plant is made available along with condition/symptom and herb(s) used is made available. No health claim has been approved by the FDA for any herbal or botanical product used as a dietary supplement to date.

Amino acids, the chief components of proteins that are the building blocks of all living structures, are divided into two categories, essential and nonessential. The eight essential amino acids plus histadine and arginine are required for health and physical well being and must be obtained from the diet whereas nonessential ones can be made by the body from other substances. Amino acid dietary supplements come in a variety of forms and also as a constituent of multiple vitamin/mineral preparations.

Health claims, if any, for both herbal/botanical and amino acid dietary supplements have not been evaluated by the FDA. Owing not only to the vast numbers of such products and the lack of useful information on them regarding their efficacy, side effects, and safety, they will not be considered further in this book. Interested readers should consult the Author's List/Web Resources, the manufacturer or distributor, and their healthcare provider for information on herbal/botanical, amino acid and other supplements.

5.10 Potential Health Benefits

Certain health claims have been FDA approved for dietary supplements. Among them are:

- calcium in the prevention/treatment of osteoporosis

- folate in the prevention of neural tube defects

- soluble fiber from whole oats and psyllium husks in the reduction of blood cholesterol (fat) levels and the prevention of coronary heart disease

- specific sugar alcohols in the prevention of dental caries (cavities).

- soy products in the prevention of cardiovascular disease

- plant sterols/stanols in the prevention of cardiovascular disease

Around 50% of adults are reported to take dietary supplements to promote health and prevent disease. Some supplements that appear to have merit are discussed in sections 5.10.1-5.10.15 respectively.

5.10.1 Fish/Flaxseed/Oils

Consuming fish/flaxseed/oils may decrease the risk of certain cancers and cardiovascular disease, and deserve consideration as supplements for these potential benefits. For additional information on fish/fish oils, see section 1.10, and for flaxseed/flaxseed oils, see section 1.11.

5.10.2 Niacin

High doses of niacin (greater than 1,000 milligrams per day) may reduce levels of blood lipids/cholesterol. However, at these high levels, niacin is considered to be a drug and not a supplement, and needs to be taken under a doctor's direct supervision. It may cause serious side effects and toxicity at these higher levels, especially in susceptible individuals. See section 6.3.6 for additional information.

5.10.3 Stress Tabs

Studies have demonstrated a decreased risk of heart disease among individuals consuming higher levels of B-complex vitamins either via their diet or as a supplement. Also, alcohol consumption and the stresses of "every day living" in Western society appear to increase the need for B-complex vitamins and vitamin C. Therefore, a supplement of B-complex vitamins plus vitamin C may be useful in such cases.

5.10.4 Antioxidants/Vitamins

Fruits and vegetables are reported to help prevent a number of chronic diseases by providing antioxidants. While it is important to consume at least 5-9 servings of fruits and vegetables each day, around 75% of the population fail to do so, and thus may be deficient in antioxidants in the diet. Such antioxidants as vitamins C and E, and the carotenoids including beta carotene, lycopene, and lutein are regarded by many as protective of healthy cells in the body from damage caused by free radicals, and thus help prevent the onset of chronic diseases.

Men with the lowest levels of beta carotene, for example, are reported to have the greatest risk of developing prostate cancer. See section 6.2.1 for additional information.

Lycopene is reported to protect against cardiovascular disease and cancer of the colon, esophagus, mouth, pharnyx, prostate, stomach and rectum. Women with the highest levels of lycopene in their blood are reported to be 5 times less likely to develop precancerous cervical lesions.

Lutein also is reported to protect against heart attacks and stroke. Individuals with the lowest blood levels of lutein show the most carotid artery thickening, a potential precursor for stroke. In addition, lutein is reported to reduce the risk of age related macular degeneration, a major cause of blindness in the elderly.

Vitamin E is reported to affect athletic performance, aging, cancer, cataracts, infertility, heart disease and mental/cognitive decline in the elderly. It may even modestly slow the progression of Alzheimer's disease. See section 6.2.3 for additional information.

Vitamin C is reported to lower blood pressure and cholesterol levels, and prevent heart attacks and stroke. Risk of stroke is reported to be 2-3 times higher in men with low blood vitamin C levels. Overweight men, those with high blood pressure, or with low blood levels of vitamin C, are reported to have 3 times higher risk of stroke. Vitamin C may also play a role in improving lung function and decreasing wheezing in patients with asthma, chronic bronchitis, and emphysema. It also may offer some protection against the adverse effects of atmospheric pollution and smoking. See section 6.3.1 for additional information.

Food is still considered the best source of antioxidant vitamins and minerals. However, certain persons commonly don't receive all of the antioxidant vitamins/minerals needed from food for a variety of reasons. They may smoke, consume too much alcohol, or don't eat the right variety of foods. Lack of appetite, decreased sense of taste or smell and depression in the elderly also can contribute to poor nutrition and deficiencies in essential antioxidant vitamins and minerals. Thus, for such persons and those on restrictive diets for a variety of conditions and reasons, supplements may be necessary and useful. Because such diets often are deficient in more than one vitamin and/or mineral, a multivitamin/mineral supplement makes more sense for most adults rather than a single nutrient supplement unless only a single nutrient deficiency state is demonstrated to exist.

5.10.5 Vitamin D

Up to 50-60% of all adults admitted to a hospital are reported to have blood levels of vitamin D that are insufficient for maintaining bone density and avoiding fractures. Deficiency of vitamin D, in terms of low blood levels of the vitamin, may even be found in up to 40% of individuals who consume more than the recommended amount of vitamin D from either diet or who take a multivitamin supplement. This suggests that current recommended intake for vitamin D may be too low, especially for individuals who live in the northern parts of the US and don't produce enough vitamin D, especially during the winter months, due to lack of exposure to the sun and the fact that the sun's rays are too weak during this time of the year. Also, milk and its products fortified with vitamin D not uncommonly do not contain consistent amounts of the vitamin, perhaps in as much as 50% of samples tested. Studies indicate that supplemental doses of vitamin D in the elderly may reduce total fracture rate by at least 20%, and fractures in osteoporotic bone sites by at least 30%. Low blood levels of vitamin D also have been associated with increased risk of heart attacks. Individuals over the age of 65 who have used vitamin D supplements are reported to have a 30% less risk of heart disease. Therefore, individuals who may be at high risk for vitamin D deficiency should consider vitamin

D supplements under the supervision of a doctor. See section 6.2.2 for additional information.

5.10.6 Folate

Homocysteine blood levels are reported to be higher in elderly individuals with low intake of B vitamins, especially folate. Research indicates that homocysteine, a byproduct of our own amino acid metabolism, increases the risk of heart attacks and stroke, and may play a role in Alzheimer's disease and poor cognitive function in the elderly with and without dementia. Up to 75% of dementia in the elderly may be due to stroke or Alzheimer's disease. While folate usually lowers homocysteine levels, it also appears to protect the elderly from memory loss even if homocysteine levels remain high. While all grain products have been fortified with folate since 1998, additional supplemental intake may be considered in order to bring total intake up to 800 micrograms per day in the elderly. See section 6.3.9 for additional information.

5.10.7 Vitamin B-12

A recent study of Americans, aged 26 to 83, found that almost 20% were deficient in vitamin B-12, and memory loss can be one of the first symptoms of such a deficiency. In contrast, among those who took a multivitamin which contained B-12, only around 8% were found to be deficient. See section 6.3.10 for additional information.

5.10.8 Garlic

Epidemiological data indicate that individuals who consume increased amounts of garlic and other alliums have a lower risk of developing stomach cancer. Those taking 600-1000 mg of garlic per day as a supplement (equivalent to about one clove), are reported to have 8-10% lower total blood cholesterol levels. Laboratory studies suggest that garlic also regulates the production of nitric acid, a substance that helps control blood pressure by relaxing blood vessel walls. There is a blood clotting inhibiting substance in garlic called ajoene that may protect against heart attacks and stroke. Raw rather than cooked garlic is recommended for these effects since cooking heat tends to destroy the enzyme involved in its production. For those who cannot tolerate fresh garlic or don't desire "bad breath" from eating raw garlic, supplements are considered a reasonable alternative. A report on "Garlic and Cancer Prevention" is available at:

http://www.cancer.gov/nescenter/pressreleases/garlic

5.10.9 Chromium

Some research indicates that doses up to 400 micrograms per day of chromium may be effective in lowering blood sugar levels in diabetics. While this dosage level is some 3 times or more the recommended daily intake of 120 micrograms per day, it is still well under the safe upper level of intake (UL) of 1,000 micrograms pre day. Therefore, chromium supplements may be considered in select, difficult to manage cases of diabetes mellitus (non-insulin-dependent type 2) under the direct supervision of a physician. See chapter 6.6.1 for additional information.

5.10.10 Magnesium

Diabetes is commonly associated with low magnesium blood levels, and one out of every three diabetics have such low levels. Research also indicates that as magnesium intake increases, the risk of developing non-insulin-dependent type 2 diabetes goes down. Magnesium supplements are reported to improve insulin resistance and blood sugar control and may be considered under the direct supervision of a doctor. Patients with high blood pressure and chronic congestive heart failure also not uncommonly benefit from magnesium supplementation in the diet as well. See section 6.4.2 for additional information.

5.10.11 Potassium

Insufficient intake of potassium in the diet may raise the risk of hypertension and stroke by as much as 50%. Recommended daily intake for potassium is 3,500 milligrams but many individuals often do not reach this goal. If for any reason, dietary intake does not provide this recommended amount, a potassium supplement may be considered under the direct supervision of a physician. See section 6.5.2 for additional information.

5.10.12 Calcium

Calcium in milk (300 mg per cup), fortified cereal (up to 250 mg per serving) and fortified orange juice (300 to 350 mg per cup) are recommended ways to increase dietary intake. However, individuals under age 50 need 1,000 mg/day, and those over 50 need 1,200 mg/day of calcium. Most people find it difficult to obtain these recommended dietary intakes and need supplements to do so. Calcium carbonate or calcium citrate supplements may be considered in order to make up the difference between dietary and total daily recommended intake. See section 6.4.1 for additional information.

5.10.13 Multivitamin/Mineral

Around 50% of Americans over the age of 50 are reported to take dietary supplements, and the supplement most often consumed is a multivitamin/mineral one formulated at 100% of the Daily Value for essential vitamins and minerals. In a 2001 study, a multivitamin/mineral supplement significantly increased blood levels of vitamins C, D, E, B-2, B-12, and folate to intake levels previously associated with reduced risk of chronic disease in older adults. Taking a standard daily multivitamin and a daily 200 IU supplement of vitamin E also is reported to reduce the risk of colon cancer by 50%. Thus, multivitamin/mineral and vitamin E supplements may be considered beneficial for adults, particularly those over the age of 50.

5.10.14 Tea

Green tea originated in Asia in ancient times, making its way to the West more recently. While the health benefits of green tea have been recognized for some time, black tea is now also being reported to share in these benefits and now accounts for most tea consumption in North America.

Tea is reported to be the most commonly consumed beverage in the world after water. All green, black, red (oolong), and white teas are derived from the leaf of the warm weather evergreen tree plant know as Camellia sinensis. Leaves of this tree, from which teas are made, contain flavonoids (otherwise known as polyphenols or catechins) which have significant antioxidant properties. Herbal teas, on the other hand, are from different plants and do not contain the health promoting flavonoids.

Processing determines whether tea will be white, green, red or black. White teas are minimally oxidized teas made from very young tea leaf buds that are not withered and are steamed immediately to prevent oxidation. Examples include Mutan White, Flowery Peking White, and White Pearls. Green teas are made from "mature" leaves and are minimally processed. Black and red teas, made from the leaf, are first partially dried, and then crushed and fermented with the length of fermentation determining whether the tea will be red (oolong) or black. Oolong teas (Cantonese, Formosa and Jade for example) are processed for shorter periods of time compared with black teas. All teas, regardless of their processing contain flavonoids, but green teas contain more than black varieties. Tea also is regarded as a significant dietary source of fluoride and manganese providing as much as 1 milligram in each 8 ounce serving.

Flavonoids in tea, like other antioxidants, are believed to protect cells from the damaging effects of "oxidative stress" and free radicals that can lead to cancer, cardiovascular disease, and other chronic conditions. A number of studies have provided evidence for the anticancer effects of the flavonoids including:

- reducing damage that free radicals may do to cells/DNA

- blocking enzymes essential for tumor growth

- deactivating cancer promoting substances.

The major flavonoids (polyphenols) in tea are the catechins. Catechins are antioxidant compounds found principally in green tea but also in significant amounts in black tea. The four principal catechins in tea include epicatechin (EC), epigallocatechin (EGC), epigallocatechin gallate (EGCG), and gallocatechin (GC). The somewhat lower amounts of these catechins in black tea may be due to the way it is processed/dried/fermented. EGCG is reported to be as much as 80-100 times more potent than vitamin C, and 20-25 times more potent than vitamin E in antioxidant activity.

Catechins appear to be important antioxidants in:

- reducing the risk of cancer and cardiovascular disease by combating lipid peroxidation and free radical damage within cell membranes and artery walls

- protecting against certain cancers by suppressing growth of tumors and inhibiting enzymes that are involved in the spread of cancer cells. EGCG appears to be unique in its ability to fight cancer at all stages, namely by:
  - inhibiting development of tumors
  - irradicating tumor promoters
  - blocking chemical carcinogens
  - neutralizing enzymes involved in cell proliferation

- providing antimicrobial activity that suppresses the growth of bacteria such as:
  - E. coli responsible for infectious diarrhea and other serious infections
  - Heliobacter pylori involved in gastrointestinal ulcers and gastric cancer
  - Staphylococcus aureus, the causative agent for common bacterial infections, both minor and serious

Steeping either green or black tea for around 5 minutes is reported to release over 80% of its catechins. Instant iced tea, on the other hand, contains negligible amounts of catechins.

A number of health benefits have been reported in individuals who drink tea. Postmenopausal women who drank at least 2 cups of black tea per day are reported to be 40% less likely to develop urinary tract cancer, and 68% less likely to suffer from cancer of the digestive tract. Other research studies indicate that drinking tea may also help prevent bladder, esophagus, lung, prostate, and stomach cancer. Among men evaluated in China, tea drinkers were found to be about half as likely to develop stomach or esophageal cancer as men who drank little or no tea. However, a similar study in the Netherlands did not support the findings.

Tea also is reported to show promise in the prevention of coronary heart disease and stroke. Individuals who drank tea are reported to be the least likely to die 3-4 years after a heart attack. Flavonoids and other substances in tea are believed to be responsible for this effect. Other research studies link moderate tea drinking with a 30% lower death rate from heart disease, heavy tea drinkers a 44% lower death rate. Flavonoids in tea inhibit the oxidation of low density lipoprotein cholesterol (LDL-C) and have an anticlotting effect (keeping blood platelets from clumping) both of which may be responsible, at least in part, for this beneficial effect. Men and women who drink more than 3-5 cups of tea daily are reported to have up to a 40% reduced risk of stroke. Blood vessel dilation is reported to be improved after drinking tea and this may account, at least in part, for the beneficial effects of tea regarding stroke and coronary heart disease.

Elderly women who drank at least one cup of tea daily are reported to have higher bone densities in the spine and hip areas, common sites for fractures due to osteoporosis.

Adding milk to tea may decrease absorption of the antioxidant flavonoids and may decrease tea's reported beneficial health effects.

Fluoride concentrations in tea are reported to be comparable to those recommended for US water supplies for the prevention of tooth decay. And tea extracts have been found to prevent dental caries in clinical trials.

Tea extracts as concentrated sources of tea flavonoids are available as dietary supplements. They may be labeled as tea catechins or tea polyphenols.

Additional information on tea and its potential health benefits are available at:
http://lpi.oregonstate.edu/infocenter/phytochemicals/tea/tea.html
http://www.webmd.com (search "tea")
http://www.cancer.gov (search "tea")

5.10.15 Plant Sterols/Stanols

The FDA has approved health claims regarding the role of plant sterol/stanol esters in reducing the risk of coronary heart disease by lowering blood cholesterol levels. Studies indicate that 1.3 grams per day of plant sterols or 3.4

grams per day of plant stanol esters are needed to show a significant cholesterol lowering effect. Plant sterols are present in small quantities in many fruits, vegetables, nuts, seeds, cereals, legumes, other plant sources, and vegetable oils. Plant stanols also occur in some of the same food sources. However, the amounts of sterol/stanol esters present in natural foods are considered to be too low to provide much health benefits. Therefore, foods and supplements have been fortified with sufficient amounts for the desired effect. Fortified foods that may qualify for the FDA health claim based on plant sterol ester content include spreads, salad dressings, and snack bars. Supplements containing at least 0.65 grams of plant sterol esters, taken twice a day with meals for a total daily intake of at least 1.3 grams, as part of a diet low in saturated fat and cholesterol may produce sufficient blood cholesterol, lowering and reduce the risk of cardiovascular disease, and qualify for this FDA approved health claim.

6. Essential Vitamins/Minerals

6.1 Introduction

Essential vitamins/minerals are substances the body requires in small amounts for normal growth, development, function and health. Because of the small amounts of each required, these substances collectively are called essential micronutrients. As the body is unable to make essential micronutrients, they must be obtained from food sources in the diet, or in some cases, from dietary or medically administered supplements. Micronutrients enable the body to process (metabolize) carbohydrates, fats and proteins for energy, growth and development, and health. While they don't provide any fuel (calories or energy) in themselves, they do help the body effectively provide and use energy (calories) from food.

Fourteen (14) vitamins currently are recognized as essential for humans. These fall into two basic categories, namely:

- Fat soluble: vitamins A, D, E and K which are stored in body fat

- Water soluble: vitamin C, biotin, choline and the seven B-vitamins, namely: B-1 (thiamine), B-2 (riboflavin), B-3 (niacin), B-5 (pantothenic acid), B-6 (pyridoxine), B-9 (folate/folic acid), and B-12 (cobalamin), which are only stored in the body in limited amounts as compared with the fat soluble vitamins.

The 14 essential vitamins are discussed in sections 6.1-6.3 respectively.

The body also requires certain key minerals for normal growth, development, function and health. These are discussed in sections 6.4-6.6.

The first group of key minerals required in the diet in amounts greater than 100 milligrams/day are referred to as major minerals. They are calcium, magnesium, and phosphorous, and are important in the development of health, bones and teeth, etc. They are discussed in section 6.4.

The mineral electrolytes, sodium, chloride, and potassium regulate fluid and mineral balance. These are discussed in section 6.5

The essential minerals needed in smaller amounts in the diet (less than 100 milligrams/day) are called trace minerals. Chromium, cobalt, copper, fluorine, iodine, iron, manganese, molybdenum, selenium and zinc fall into this group, and are discussed in section 6.6.

Another group of trace minerals has been identified, however, their status as essential needs to be clarified, and they remain unclassified. Chief among these are boron, lithium, nickel, silicon, and vanadium. Since they are not yet considered as essential, they will not be considered further in this book except for boron, discussed in section 6.7. Those desirous of more information on these minerals may obtain it from websites in the Author's List/Key Web Resources in Chapter 7.

The Recommended Dietary Allowance (RDA) also referred to as the Recommended Daily Allowance, and Daily Value (DV) should not be confused with daily nutritional requirements for an individual. RDAs were developed for healthy people living under "normal" circumstances, (e.g. no illness or excessive life "stressors"), and estimating amounts of each micronutrient necessary to prevent development of a manifest deficiency state. In addition, studies which serve as a basis for such RDAs and DVs typically involve only short periods of time (months not years), and only around 1% of the average human life span. Therefore, the amounts of nutrients, sufficient to provide continued health and prevent of disease over short periods of time, may be inadequate to maintain health over the entire life span under all possible life's conditions. Thus, RDAs and DVs are intended as a guide only.

The reader should bear in mind that definitive scientific evidence is lacking at this time to substantiate that consuming large doses (more than three times) above the Recommended Dietary Allowance (RDA) or Daily Value (DV) of any essential vitamin or mineral in the diet, or as a supplement, has any significant health benefit, except in deficiency states. Diagnosis and treatment of deficiency states requires the direct supervision of a physician.

6.2 Fat soluble Vitamins

The 4 fat soluble vitamins, A, D, E and K are discussed in 6.2.1-6.2.4 respectively.

6.2.1 Vitamin A (Retinol/Beta Carotene)

Vitamin A is a family of fat soluble vitamins with retinol being one of the most active, or usable forms. Retinol is often called preformed vitamin A. It can be converted in the body to retinol and retinoic acid, other active forms of the vitamin A family. Beta carotene is a provitamin A that is converted to retinol/vitamin A in the body. Alpha carotene is also converted to vitamin A in the body but only half as efficiently as beta carotene.

Vitamin A plays an important role in vision, bone growth, reproduction, and cell division and differentiation (a process by which a cell decides what it is going to become). It helps maintain the surface linings of the eyes, and the respiratory, urinary, and intestinal tracts. It also helps maintain the integrity of skin and mucous membranes that function as a barrier to bacteria and viruses. When such linings break down, bacteria can enter the body and cause infection. Vitamin A also helps regulate the immune system to prevent or fight off infections by making white blood cells, such as lymphocytes, more effective at destroying harmful bacteria and viruses. Some vitamin A precursors have been shown to function as antioxidants in laboratory tests. Antioxidants protect cells from free radicals which are potentially damaging byproducts of oxygen metabolism that may contribute to the development of some chronic diseases.

Preformed vitamin A is found in animal foods such as whole eggs and whole milk, liver, and fortified breakfast cereals. Provitamin A is abundant in dark colored fruits and vegetables. Most fat free milk and dried nonfat milk solids sold in the US are fortified with vitamin A to replace that which is lost when the fat is removed.

It is important to regularly eat foods that provide vitamin A or its precursors even though vitamin A is stored in the liver. Stored vitamin A helps to meet the body's needs when intake of provitamin A or preformed vitamin A are low.

There is no RDA for beta carotene or other provitamin A carotenoids. The IOM suggests consuming 3-6 mg of beta carotene will maintain plasma beta carotene blood levels in the range associated with a lower risk of chronic diseases. A diet that provides five or more servings of fruits and vegetables per day and includes dark green and leafy vegetables, and deep yellow or orange fruits should provide the recommended amounts of beta carotene.

Vitamin A deficiency:

- rarely occurs in the United States but is still a major public health problem in less developed countries.

  At least 3 million children worldwide develop xeropthalmia (damage to the cornea of each eye) and 250-500,000 go blind each year from a deficiency of vitamin A. Night blindness is one of the first signs of vitamin A deficiency which contributes to blindness by making the cornea very dry (xeropthalmia) and promoting damage to the cornea and retina.

- diminishes the ability to fight infections, especially in less developed countries.

- is especially important in countries where immunization programs are not widespread and vitamin A deficiency is common, and millions of children die each year from complications of infectious diseases. In such vitamin A deficiency cases, cells lining the lung lose their ability to remove disease causing microorganisms, contributing to pneumonia and death.

Subclinical forms (mild degrees) of vitamin A deficiency with low storage levels of vitamin A that do not cause overt deficiency symptoms, may increase children's risk of developing respiratory and diarrheal infections, decrease growth rate, slow bone development, and decrease the likelihood of survival from serious illness. Children living in the United States that are considered to be at increased risk for subclinical vitamin A deficiency include those:

- living at or below the poverty line

- with inadequate health care or immunizations

- living in areas with known nutritional deficiencies

- immigrants or refugees from developing countries with a high incidence of vitamin A deficiency or measles

- with disease of the pancreas, liver, intestines, or with inadequate fat digestion/absorption who are toddlers and preschool children.

Vitamin A deficiency in adults can occur when vitamin A is lost through chronic diarrhea, in patients with cystic fibrosis, sprue, pancreatic disorders and after gastrointestinal bypass surgery for obesity, as well as in vegetarians. Protein, calories, and zinc are needed to make retinol binding protein (RBP) which is essential for mobilizing vitamin A from the liver and transporting it to the general circulation and tissues where it may be needed.

Excess alcohol intake may deplete vitamin A stores. Also, diets high in alcohol intake generally do not provide recommended amounts of vitamin A. Anyone who consumes excessive amounts of alcohol needs to include adequate sources of vitamin A in the diet or consider vitamin A supplementation.

Vegetarians who do not consume eggs and dairy food need supplemental amounts of vitamin A in their diet. It is important for them to include a minimum of five servings of fruits and vegetables daily, and to regularly choose dark green leafy vegetables and orange and yellow fruits in order to consume the recommended amounts of vitamin A.

In women over 50 at least 3.7 milligrams of beta carotene a day from food, (about a half of a carrot), is reported to reduce the risk of breast cancer in women by around 68%.

The IOM indicates that beta carotene and vitamin A supplements usually are not advisable for the general population but may be useful for the prevention of deficiency in populations with inadequate vitamin A intake in the diet.

Hypervitaminosis A refers to high storage levels of vitamin A due to excessive intake which can lead to adverse/toxic effects such as birth defects, liver abnormalities and reduced bone mineral density that may result in osteopenia, osteoporosis, and bone fractures.

While hypervitaminosis A can occur when very large amounts of liver are regularly consumed, most cases result from an excess intake of vitamin A in supplements. The IOM has established daily tolerable upper levels (UL) of intake from supplements in adults at 10,000 IU*. Provitamin A carotenoids are generally considered to be reasonably safe because they are not usually associated with adverse effects. Also, the conversion of provitamin A carotenoids and beta carotene to vitamin A decreases significantly when body stores are full, which naturally limits further increases in storage levels. A high intake of provitamin A can turn the skin yellow, but this is not considered dangerous to health. The IOM also has not set a tolerable upper intake level (UL) for beta carotene.

* to convert IUs to milligrams multiply by 0.0006. To convert milligrams to IUs divide by 0.0006.

Additional information as well as selected food sources for vitamin A can be found at:

http://www.cc.nih.gov/ccc/supplements/vita.html

http://www.nlm.nih.gov/medlineplus (search "vitamin A")

http://www.foodstandards.gov.uk

6.2.2 Vitamin D (Calciferol)

Vitamin D, calciferol, is a fat soluble vitamin that not only is found in food, but also can be made in the body after exposure to ultraviolet rays from the sun. Vitamin D exists in several forms, each with a different activity. Some forms are relatively inactive in the body and have limited ability to function as vitamin D. The liver and kidneys help convert vitamin D to its chief active hormone form, vitamin D-3.

The major biologic function of vitamin D is to maintain normal blood and tissue levels of calcium and phosphorous. Vitamin D aids in the absorption of calcium and promotes bone mineralization in concert with other vitamins, minerals and hormones. Without vitamin D, bone becomes thin, brittle, soft and fractures more easily. It prevents rickets in children and osteomalacia in adults which are skeletal diseases that result in weakened bones.

Fortified foods are the major dietary sources of vitamin D. One cup of vitamin D fortified milk supplies about one fourth of the estimated daily need for this vitamin in adults. Products made from milk such as cheese, yogurt and ice cream generally are not fortified with vitamin D. Only a few foods, such as fatty fish and fish oils naturally contain significant amounts of vitamin D.

Exposure to sunlight is an important source of vitamin D in humans. Ultraviolet rays (UV) from sunlight trigger vitamin D synthesis in the skin. Season, latitude, time of day, cloud cover, smog and sunscreens affect UV ray exposure. In the Northeast USA the average amount of sunlight generally is insufficient to produce significant vitamin D synthesis from November to February. Sunscreens with a protection factor of 8 or greater block UV rays that produce vitamin D. Therefore, it is especially important for individuals with limited sun exposure to include good food sources of vitamin D in their diet.

A deficiency of vitamin D can occur when dietary intake is inadequate or exposure to sunlight is limited, as well as when the kidneys and/or liver cannot convert vitamin D to its active form, calcitriol, and when someone cannot adequately absorb dietary vitamin D. Classic vitamin D deficiency diseases are rickets, (skeletal deformities in children) and osteomalacia (muscular and bone "weakness" in adults).

Older Americans (greater than age 50) are regarded as having a higher risk of developing vitamin D deficiency. The ability of skin and kidneys to convert vitamin D to its active form decreases with age. Kidneys sometimes do not work as well due to disease as people age. Therefore, some older Americans may need added vitamin D as a supplement. Having normal storage levels of vitamin D helps prevent osteoporosis in the elderly, nonambulatory individuals, post menopausal women, and those on chronic steroid therapy.

A recent study of patients admitted to hospital showed that 57% had vitamin D blood levels low enough to be regarded as deficient. Even more alarming, 46% were deficient even if they took a daily multivitamin containing the recommended DV of 400 I.U. of vitamin D (10 micrograms).

Individuals with limited sun exposure, homebound persons, people living in northern latitudes, such as New England and Alaska, women who cover their face and bodies for religious reasons, and those working in occupations that prevent exposure to sunlight, are at risk of a vitamin D deficiency. If these individuals are unable to meet their dietary need for vitamin D, a supplement may be needed.

Those who have reduced ability to absorb dietary fat also may need extra vitamin D because it requires fat in the diet for satisfactory absorption. Malabsorption of vitamin D may occur in pancreatic enzyme deficiency, Crohn's disease, cystic fibrosis, sprue, liver disease, gastric bypass surgery for obesity, and small bowel disease. Diarrhea and greasy stools are characteristic symptoms of fat malabsorption.

A significant health risk is associated with consuming too much vitamin D. Toxicity may produce nausea, vomiting, poor appetite, constipation, weakness, and weight loss. Increased blood levels of calcium may cause mental status changes such as confusion, and abnormalities of heart rhythm. Deposition of calcium and phosphate in soft tissues like the kidneys also can occur. However, consuming too much vitamin D through diet alone is not very likely unless one routinely consumes large amounts of cod liver oil. Adverse effects/toxicity is more likely to result from high intakes of vitamin D via supplements.

The IOM has established a safe, tolerable upper limit (UL) for adult males and females at 50 micrograms (2,000 IU/day). Daily intakes above this level may increase the risk of adverse effects and should be avoided.

Additional vitamin D information and selected food sources are available at:
http://www.cc.nih.gov/supplements/vitd.html
http://www.nlm.nih.gov/medlineplus (search "vitamin D")
http://www.foodstandard.gov.uk

6.2.3 Vitamin E (Tocopherols)

Vitamin E (tocopherols) exists in several different forms. Each form has its own biological activity. Alpha tocopherol is the most active form. It is a powerful antioxidant that protects cells against the effects of free radicals that may contribute to the development of cardiovascular disease and cancer. Vegetable oils, nuts, green leafy vegetable and fortified cereals are the main dietary sources of vitamin E.

Deficiency is rare in adults except in persons who cannot absorb dietary fat (e.g. cystic fibrosis, Crohn's disease, etc.) and those with rare disorders of fat metabolism. A vitamin E deficiency may be characterized by neurological problems due to poor nerve conduction.

Vitamin E may help prevent or delay coronary heart disease and the formation of blood clots which could lead to a heart attack or stroke. Lower heart disease risk is associated with higher vitamin E intake (e.g. 400-800 IU). However, not all studies have provided evidence of vitamin E efficacy in the prevention or treatment of cardiovascular disease or stroke. The HOPE (Heart Outcomes Prevention Evaluation) study found that giving 400 IU of natural vitamin E per day for 4.5 years to people with heart disease did not reduce their risk of having a heart attack or stroke. Also, an Italian study found that giving 300 IU of synthetic E a day for 3.5 years did not offer any protection against heart attacks. However, other studies appear to show that vitamin E may prevent heart disease. In two such studies, a group from the Harvard School of Public Health found that individuals who took at least 100 I.U. of vitamin E a day for at least 2 years had about a 40% lower risk of heart disease. In addition other research indicates that vitamin E reduces low density lipoprotein oxidation, and blocks clotting factors that can lead to a heart attack.

Antioxidants such as vitamin E also are believed to help protect against the damaging effects of free radicals that may contribute to the development of cancer and other chronic diseases. Vitamin E also blocks the formation of nitrosamines, cancer causing carcinogens formed in the gastrointestinal tract from nitrates consumed in the diet. And, vitamin E may protect against the development of cancers by enhancing immune function.

A higher intake of vitamin E is associated with a decreased incidence of prostate, breast, and colon cancers. A study of diets of 64 hospitalized patients found that men with the highest intake of vitamin E had about a 75% lower risk of intestinal adenomas (a precursor of colon cancer). However, evidence is insufficient to recommend vitamin E supplements for the prevention of colon cancer.

Some studies have found that lens clarity, used to diagnose cataracts, was better in regular users of vitamin E supplements and in individuals with higher blood levels of vitamin E. As a result, antioxidants also are being studied to determine whether they can help prevent or delay cataract formation.

The health risk of too much vitamin E appears to be low. Vitamin E supplements for up to four months, at doses up to 800 IU have been reported to have no significant adverse effect on general health. The IOM has set an upper tolerable intake (UL) vitamin E at 1,500 IU for any form of supplementary vitamin E per day because this nutrient can act as an anticoagulant and increase the risk of bleeding problems. The UL represents the maximum intake of a nutrient that is likely to pose little or no risk of adverse health effects in most, but not all, individuals.

Diabetics with poor control and high blood sugar levels generate an overabundance of free radicals. Vitamin E supplements are reported to reduce such free radical production that may lead to damaged arteries and cardiovascular disease. Also, 800 I.U. of vitamin E daily is reported to reduce blood sugar levels significantly in diabetics.

Vitamin E also appears to enhance immune function, particularly in the elderly. A daily dose of 800 I.U. of vitamin E is reported to enhance immune responsiveness (T-cell function) which is reported to play a role in warding off infections and cancer.

Available evidence indicates that individuals may protect their health without harmful side effects by taking a daily vitamin E supplement of around 400-800 I.U. in consultation with a doctor. It generally is not feasible to obtain these high levels of intake of vitamin E from foods alone since this would entail excessive fat/caloric intake to do so.

Additional vitamin E information and selected food sources are available at:
http://www.cc.nih.gov/ccc/supplements/vite.html
http://www.nlm.nih.gov/medlineplus (search "vitamin E")
http://www.foodstandards.gov.uk

6.2.4 Vitamin K (phylloquinone)

Vitamin K (phylloquinone) is an essential fat soluble vitamin known to play a principal role in blood clotting. More recent studies indicate that it also is important in maintaining strong bones, particularly in the elderly.

There are two basic forms of vitamin K, phylloquinone, or vitamin K-1 found in food, and menaquinone, or vitamin K-2 produced by bacteria in the intestines. Both forms appear to be adequately absorbed from the intestine. However, there is little storage of vitamin K in the body. Limited stores, mainly in the liver, are only slowly utilized.

Recent evidence suggests that the current RDA/DV may not be sufficient for maximizing vitamin K's function(s) in bones. The amount of vitamin K needed to optimize the modification of osteocalcin and other proteins that build and maintain bone calcification/strength needs further clarification. However, vitamin K adds carboxyl groups to osteocalcin and other proteins that build and maintain bone. To be fully active, the bone building protein osteocalcin needs to be saturated with carboxyl groups. Vitamin K is considered to have a protective effect against bone fractures. Hip fractures in particular, appear to be associated with lower blood levels of vitamin K and saturation levels of osteocalcin.

Food sources for vitamin K include brussels sprouts, broccoli, cabbage, cauliflower, collards, kale, spinach, swiss chard, and other green leafy vegetables. Whole grain cereals, soybeans, oils, and other vegetables also serve as food sources for vitamin K. Bacteria found in the intestines also produce vitamin K for absorption and use by the body. However, dark green vegetables provide most of the vitamin K needed for health.

Significant numbers of individuals consume another form of vitamin K known as dihydrophylloquinone that is produced during the processing and hydrogenation of vegetable oils. About half of the US soybean oil is hydrogenated. The degree of hydrogenation ranges from light, for margarines, spreads, and cooking oils used in restaurants, to heavy, for deep frying and bakery products. As much as 30% of the total vitamin K intake in the U.S. may come in the form of dihydrophylloquinone which is only half as active regarding clot forming protein and completely inactive concerning bone forming protein. Therefore, hydrogenated oils should not be considered an important source of vitamin K in the diet.

Three major causes of vitamin K deficiency exist, namely: inadequate dietary intake, intestinal malabsorption, and loss of storage sites due to hepatocellular (liver) disease. Vitamin K deficiency is rare and usually occurs when there is an inability to absorb the vitamin from the intestinal tract. Deficiency can also occur after prolonged treatment with broad spectrum antibiotics that suppress bacterial production of vitamin K in the intestine. Individuals with vitamin K deficiency usually have an increased propensity to easy bruising and bleeding (e.g. gastrointestinal bleeding, coughing up blood, blood in the urine, and post operative hemorrhage). People taking warfarin (a blood thinner) should be aware that vitamin K, or foods containing vitamin K, may interfere with the effectiveness of this medication.

Individuals hospitalized in tertiary care centers commonly exhibit subtle vitamin K deficiency, with blood levels of vitamin K below mean levels for healthy adults. As vitamin K is now considered to be necessary for the syntheses of proteins involved in normal bone growth and maintenance, subtle vitamin K deficiency may be a contributing factor in fractures. This suggests that vitamin K supplementation should be considered in such patients.

Vitamin K appears to be nontoxic to animals, even when given in large amounts. Intravenous administration of phylloquinone has been reported to produce flushing, shortness of breath, chest pains, cardiovascular collapse, and rarely death. Menadione (K-3) is irritating to the skin and respiratory tract. In patients who have liver disease, vitamin K may further depress liver function.

Deficiency of vitamin K is best established and treated by a physician. Various dietary interventions and vitamin K supplementation regimens are available for these purposes.

Additional vitamin K information and selected food sources are available at:
http://www.nlm.nih.gov/medlineplus (search "vitamin K")
http://www.foodstandards.gov.uk

6.3 Water soluble Vitamins

The 10 water soluble vitamins are discussed in sections 6.3.1-6.3.10 respectively.

6.3.1 Vitamin C (Ascorbic Acid)

Vitamin C, an essential water soluble vitamin, is also known as ascorbic acid. It is required for the:

- synthesis of collagen, an important structural component of blood vessels, tendons, ligaments, bone and skin,

- production of the neurotransmitters like norepinephrine, that can affect brain function, mood, etc.,

- synthesis of carnitine which is essential for the transport of fat to cellular organelles called mitochondria for conversion to energy,

- metabolism of cholesterol and bile acids which may have implications for blood cholesterol levels and gallstones,

- cellular protection, as an antioxidant, of certain indispensable substances in the body, such as proteins, fats, carbohydrates, DNA, and RNA, from damage by free radicals and reactive oxygen chemicals that can be generated during normal metabolism as well as through exposure to toxins and pollutants (e.g. smoking).

- regeneration of other antioxidants such as vitamin E. Vitamin C also aids in the absorption of iron. It is a highly effective antioxidant, even small amounts can protect indispensable substances in the body.

Scurvy is the potentially fatal disease that occurs as a result of severe vitamin C deficiency. Symptoms may include fatigue, bleeding, bruising easily, hair and tooth loss, joint pain and swelling related to the weakening of blood vessels, connective tissue and bone all of which contain collagen. Fatigue may result from diminished levels of carnitine, needed to obtain energy from fat or from a decrease in the synthesis of the neurotransmitter, norepinephrine. Frank scurvy is rare in developed countries because it can be prevented by as little as 10 mg of vitamin C daily. Less severe forms of vitamin C deficiencies can also occur.

The amounts of vitamin C required to prevent chronic disease appear to be much greater than that needed for the prevention of scurvy. A number of clinical studies have demonstrated that higher levels of vitamin C intake are associated with a lower risk of heart disease and stroke, and blood levels of vitamin C are highly correlated with fruit and vegetable intake. For example, the risk of stroke in individuals who consumed fruits and vegetables 6 to 7 days of the week is reported to be only 58% of those who ate them 2 days or less per week.

Many studies have shown that increased intake of fresh fruits and vegetables is associated with a reduced risk of most types of cancer. Significant cancer risk reductions are reported to occur in individuals consuming at least 80-110 mg vitamin C daily.

Decreased vitamin C levels in the lens of the eye are associated with increased severity of cataracts in humans. Increased dietary vitamin C intake and corresponding increased blood levels of vitamin C are associated with decreased risk of cataracts. These studies suggest that vitamin C intake may have to be higher than 300 mg/day for a number of years before a protective effect against cataracts can occur. However, not all studies show a relationship between vitamin C intake and the development of cataracts, and further studies are needed to clarify the relationship.

Several studies also have demonstrated a blood pressure lowering effect when 500 mg of vitamin C supplementation are given daily to patients with high blood pressure.

A study at the National Institutes of Health found that at least 200 milligrams of vitamin C are needed to keep blood at the 85% vitamin C saturation level. For 95% saturation, we need 400 to 500 milligrams of vitamin C daily. Thus, recommended intake of vitamin C may be too low for optimum health benefits.

Clinical evidence from well controlled trials indicating that high doses of vitamin C affects the survival of cancer patients is lacking.

Eating a variety of fruits and vegetables that contain vitamin C is regarded the best way to obtain 100% of the Daily Value. Different fruits and vegetables vary in their vitamin C content but 5 to 9 servings a day should average out to around 200 mg of vitamin C daily. The amount of vitamin C depends not only on the food source but also on serving size consumed.

Foods high in vitamin C include:

Food	Vitamin C in milligrams
one guava	165
one sweet red pepper	140
cup fresh-squeezed orange juice	125
cup cranberry juice cocktail	100
cup orange juice from concentrate	95
cup strawberries	85
cup grapefruit juice from concentrate	80
cup raw broccoli	80
one kiwi	75
one orange	70
one cup canteloupe cubes	65
one sweet green pepper	65
cup pineapple	60
one mango	55
cup raw cauliflower	45
½ grapefruit	40

Vitamin C can be lost from foods during preparation, cooking or storage. To help maximize vitamin C intake:

- use an airtight container to store raw fruits and vegetables and refrigerate

- do not soak or store foods in water as vitamin C will be dissolved in the water and lost to the food

- steam, boil, or simmer foods in a minimal amount of water, or microwave for the shortest time possible

- refrigerate prepared juices and do not store them for more than 2 to 3 days

- cook potatoes in their skins.

Some juices such as grape and apple have vitamin C added. A ¾ cup serving of such fortified juice may provide up to 40 to 50% of the Daily Value for vitamin C. Fortified ready-to-eat cereals usually contain at least 25% of the RDA for vitamin C.

Supplemental vitamin C is available in a number of forms but there is little scientific evidence that any one form is better absorbed or more effective than any other. Natural and synthetic vitamin C are identical and there are no known differences in their bioavailability or biological activities.

The safe tolerable upper limit (UL) of vitamin C is set at 2,000 mg/day by IOM. Doses below this UL prevent most adults from experiencing diarrhea and other gastrointestinal disturbances that may occur at higher doses.

Additional vitamin C information and selected food sources are available at:
http://lpi.oregonstate.edu/infocenter/vitamins/vitaminC/c.html
http://www.nlm.nih.gov/medlineplus (search "vitamin C")
http://www.foodstandards.gov.uk

6.3.2 Biotin

Biotin is a water soluble essential B-complex vitamin. Bacteria that normally colonize the large intestine are capable of synthesizing biotin and humans may absorb significant amounts of biotin made by intestinal bacteria. Biotin functions as a cofactor in the body's key enzyme systems called carboxylases and catatalyzes essential metabolic reactions involving:

- synthesis of fatty acids

- formation of glucose from sources other than carbohydrates (e.g. amino acids and fats)

- metabolism of leucine, an essential amino acid

- metabolism of other amino acids, cholesterol and fatty acids

Biotin is found in many foods. Wheat bran, egg yolk, liver and yeast are rich sources of this vitamin. National survey data estimate average daily dietary intake of biotin to be in the range of 40-60 micrograms per day.

Deficiency is rare in humans but may occur under at least four conditions, namely:

- prolonged consumption of raw egg white which binds biotin in the gut and prevents adequate absorption

- total parenteral nutrition without biotin supplementation

- malabsorption disorders such as sprue and celiac disease

- hereditary carboxylase enzyme deficiency states

Also, individuals on long-term anticonvulsant therapy have been found to have reduced levels of biotin in their blood and decreased carboxylase enzyme activity in the body. Some anticonvulsants such as primidone and carbamazepin inhibit biotin absorption in the small intestine. Long-term treatment with sulfa drugs or other antibiotics may decrease bacterial synthesis and absorption of biotin. Large doses of pantothenic acid (vitamin B-5) may compete with biotin absorption in the intestine because of similar chemical structure. All these factors may potentially increase the chances for biotin deficiency and increase the requirement for additional dietary biotin or supplementation.

Symptoms of biotin deficiency may include hair loss and a scaly red rash around the eyes, mouth, nose ("biotin facies"), and the genital area. Depression, lethargy, hallucinations, and numbness and tingling of the extremities may occur. Impaired immune function and increased susceptibility to bacterial and fungal infections have been reported in hereditary disorders of biotin metabolism.

Biotin deficiency also may result in impairment in glucose utilization. Biotin levels are reported to be significantly reduced in patients with diabetes mellitus, and lower fasting blood glucose levels are correlated with higher biotin levels. Doses of 15 to 20 milligrams of biotin daily have been found to decrease fasting blood sugar levels some 40 to 50% after 1 month in diabetics. Further studies are needed to clarify the role of biotin supplementation in the treatment of diabetes mellitus.

Biotin is reasonably well tolerated orally. Toxicity has not been reported with daily doses up to 200 milligrams used to treat hereditary biotin deficiency. A safe upper level of intake (UL) level has not been established for biotin because of lack of sufficient evidence to do so.

Additional biotin information and selected food sources are available at:
http://lpi.oregonstate.edu/infocenter/vitamins/biotin/biotin.html
http://www.nlm.nih.gov/medlineplus (search "biotin")
http://www.foodstandards.gov.uk

6.3.3 Choline

Choline is considered an essential nutrient although it is not a vitamin by strict definition (even though it was originally identified as part of the vitamin B complex). Nevertheless, it is included here for completeness.

While humans can make small amounts of choline, it must be consumed in additional amounts in the diet to maintain health. Choline is synthesized in small amounts in the body by converting the phospholipid, phosphatidylethanolamine, to phosphatidylcholine (lecithin) which, in turn, provides the choline. However, humans cannot make enough in this way to satisfy their metabolic needs, and choline intake needs to be provided primarily by dietary sources.

Choline, and substances derived from choline in the body, are involved in a number of key biological functions such as:

• cell membrane structure, integrity and signaling.

  Choline is used in the synthesis of phospholipids, phosphatidycholine, and sphinogomyelin, key structural components of all human cell membranes. Also, choline containing molecules and metabolites are known to be important in cell signaling.

- lipid transport and metabolism.

Phosphatidylcholine is required to prevent cholesterol and other fats from accumulating in and damaging the liver.

- nerve impulse transmission.

Choline is a precursor of acetylcholine, a neurotransmitter involved in muscle contraction and memory.

- production of betaine.

This substance is a major source of methyl (CH3) groups used in metabolism, such as in the conversion of homocysteine to methionine.

- regulation of homocysteine levels, a risk factor for heart disease.

Information on the choline content of various foods is spotty, and accurate levels are not readily available. Choline is mostly available in the form of the phosphatidylcholine (lecithin) content which is only around 13% choline by weight (around 4.2 grams of phosphitidylcholine provides about 550 milligrams of choline). Eggs, liver, beef, cauliflower, and peanuts/peanut butter are reasonably good sources of choline. Strict vegetarians who consume no beef, liver, or eggs may be at risk of inadequate choline intake and deficiency. A safe, tolerable upper intake level (UL) at 3.5 grams/day for adult males and females has been established.

High doses (7.5 grams/day) of choline have been reported to produce a hypotensive effect (lowering of blood pressure) which may result in dizziness and fainting. Up to 10-16 grams/day of choline may cause a "fishy" body odor (due to the production and excretion of trimethylamine), nausea, vomiting, salivation, and sweating.

Very little is known about the amount of dietary and/or supplemental choline that may be necessary to promote optimum health or prevent chronic disease in humans. Clinical research to date has not provided any convincing evidence for a beneficial effect of choline in the prevention or treatment of cancer, cardiovascular disease, memory loss, dementia, Alzheimer's disease, or any other chronic disease.

Individuals deficient in choline have developed signs of liver damage which resolved when adequate choline was provided in the diet. Choline is required to form the phosphatidylcholine portion of very low density lipoprotein particles (VLDL) which transport fat from the liver to the tissues for storage and production of energy. Choline deficiency results in inadequate amounts of VLDL being made and fat accumulation in the liver with resulting organ damage. Also, individuals fed a choline deficient diet develop elevated blood levels of an enzyme, alanine aminotransferase, indicating the presence of liver damage. Liver cells in tissue culture exhibit a process of programmed cell death (apoptosis) when deprived of choline. Choline deficient animals also exhibit fat accumulation in the liver, cirrhosis, an increased incidence of heptaocellular carcinoma, hemorrhagic kidney disease, and poor motor coordination.

Patients taking methrotrexate may require increased choline intake in the diet or as a supplement to prevent deficiency. Methotrexate, an antimetabolite drug, is used in the treatment of cancer, psoriasis, and rheumatoid arthritis. It inhibits an enzyme system, dihydrofolate reductase, and limits the availability of methyl groups and the methylation process in metabolism of cells. As a result, methotrexate may produce a diminished choline nutritional status including fatty infiltration of the liver, which can be reversed by choline supplementation.

Choline salts (bitartrate and chloride) are available for use as supplements. Phosphatidylcholine supplements also provide choline. The chemical term lecithin is synonymous with phosphatidylcholine. However, lecithin supplements may vary from 20 to 90% in their phosphatidylcholine content, and corresponding choline content.

Additional choline information including selected dietary food sources may be found at:
http://lpi.oregonstate.edu/infocenter/othernuts/choline/choline.html
http://www.nlm.nih.gov/medlineplus (search "choline")
http://www.foodstandards.gov.uk

6.3 4 Vitamin B-1 (Thiamine)

Thiamine is a water soluble, essential B-complex vitamin, also known as vitamin B-1. It occurs in the body as free thiamine and is phosphorylated to the thiamine monophosphate (TMP), thiamine triphosphate (TTP) and thiamine pyrophosphate (TPP) all of which serve as coenzymes for key enzyme functions producing energy from food. It also serves non coenzyme functions such as the flow of sodium and potassium in and out of nerve and muscle cells, and plays a role in nerve impulse conduction and voluntary muscle action.

Beriberi is the disorder that results from thiamine deficiency, affecting the cardiovascular, gastrointestinal, muscular, and nervous systems, producing cerebral, dry and wet forms of beriberi. Cerebral beriberi leads to Wernicke's encephalopathy and Korsakoff's psychosis. Wernicke's involves abnormal eye movements, stance and gait abnormalities, and disturbances in mental function. Korsakoff's involves amnesia and psychosis. Dry beriberi is characterized by a peripheral neuropathy with the "burning feet" syndrome, exaggerated reflexes, weakness of the arms and legs including diminished sensation. Muscle pain and tenderness and difficulty arising from a squatting position may also occur. Wet beriberi includes enlargement of the heart, rapid pulse, severe swelling of the legs, difficulty in breathing and congestive heart failure along with neurological symptoms.

Alcoholism associated with malnutrition is the primary cause of thiamine deficiency in industrialized countries. Deficiency may also occur in low income populations whose diets are high in carbohydrate and low in thiamine. Certain conditions such as strenuous physical exertion, fever, adolescent growth, pregnancy and breast feeding may place an individual with marginal thiamine intake at risk for developing symptomatic thiamine deficiency. HIV-infected individuals also are at increased deficiency risk. Individuals on hemodialysis lose thiamine at an increased rate putting them at risk. Diuretics also may produce increased excretion and loss of thiamine in the urine and provoke deficiency, especially in individuals with a low dietary thiamine intake. Antithiamine factor (ATF) in plants reacts with thiamine to form an inactive byproduct. Ingesting large amounts of tea or coffee containing ATF may produce thiamine deficiency. Individual's habitually consuming raw freshwater fish and raw shellfish are at higher risk of thiamine deficiency because these foods contain an enzyme, thiaminase, which inactivates the vitamin (normally thiaminase itself is inactivated by heat in cooking).

Since thiamine deficiency may produce a form of dementia, thiamine supplements have been evaluated in patients with Alzheimer's disease, however, without much success. A recent review of well controlled trials of thiamine in patients with dementia of the Alzheimer's variety, indicates no significant benefit from thiamine supplementation in doses up to 3 grams per day over a 12 month period of time.

As thiamine deficiency can lead to heart failure, a number of small short term studies have addressed the role of thiamine in congestive heart failure (CHF). These studies suggest that thiamine in doses of 200 mg/day, orally or by injection, may improve left ventricular ejection fraction (LVEF) in patients with chronic congestive heart failure. However, conclusions that can be reached from these studies are limited because of their small size, limited treatment periods, and inadequate design. Further well controlled, longer term studies are needed to assess the role of thiamine supplementation in the treatment of CHF.

Some cancer patients with rapidly growing tumors develop thiamine deficiency. As a result, some doctors use thiamine supplements to prevent such deficiencies. Others refrain from using thiamine supplements in such patients on the grounds that such may fuel the growth of very malignant tumors, and thus reserve thiamine supplementation for those cancer patients that are actually thiamine deficient. Insufficient evidence now exists to support or refute either position in the matter. Use of thiamine supplements in cancer patients should occur only under the supervision of a doctor.

A varied diet provides most healthy individuals with adequate thiamine intake to prevent deficiencies. However, institutionalization and poverty may increase the likelihood of inadequate thiamine intake, particularly in the elderly, and require supplementation.

Anticonvulsant medication, used for epilepsy, and 5-fluorouracil for cancer therapy, inhibit the phosphorylation of thiamine to TPP and thus decrease thiamine activity. Diuretics, especially furosemide (Lasix), may increase thiamine loss in the urine. These medications may result in thiamine deficiency in susceptible individuals.

Adverse thiamine effects (from foods and supplements in doses up to 200 mg/ day) are essentially unknown. The IOM has not set a safe, tolerable upper limit (UL) for thiamine.

Additional thiamine information and food sources are available at:
http://lpi.oregonstate.edu/infocenter/vitamins/thiamin/thiamin.html
http://www.nlm.nih.gov/medlineplus (search "thiamine")
http://www.foodstandards.gov.uk

6.3.5 Vitamin B-2 (Riboflavin)

Riboflavin is a water soluble B complex vitamin, also known as vitamin B-2. It is an integral part of the coenzymes FAD (flavin adenine dinucleotide) and FMN (flavin mononucleotide), collectively called flavins. Enzymes that have a flavin coenzyme are called flavoproteins. It is poorly absorbed from the intestinal tract. Only about 25% of a given amount is absorbed orally.

Individuals derive most of their energy from oxidation/reduction (redox) metabolic reactions involving the transfer of electrons. Flavins (essential for the metabolism of carbohydrates, fats and proteins) are part of this electron transport system or "respiratory chain", that is key to the body's energy production as well as the metabolism and detoxification of drugs and toxins.

Riboflavin performs key antioxidant functions in the body via gutathione (reductase and peroxidase) and uric acid (xanthine oxidase) enzyme systems. Gutathione and uric acid are regarded as among the most effective water soluble antioxidants in blood. Flavoproteins also are involved in the metabolism of other vitamins (such as vitamin B-6, folic acid and niacin) as well as in other complex nutrient interactions.

Improving riboflavin nutritional status is reported to increase circulatory hemoglobin levels. Correction of riboflavin deficiency in individuals who are both riboflavin and iron deficient improves the response of iron deficiency anemia to iron therapy.

Deficiency of riboflavin is known as ariboflavinosis. It is only rarely found in isolation. Rather it usually occurs in combination with deficiencies of other water soluble vitamins, and may be characterized by:

- anemia

- cheliosis (cracks or sores at the angles of the mouth)

- edema (swelling) of oral mucous membranes

- seborrheic dermatitis (moist, scaly skin inflammation)

- sore throat (painful reddish inflammation of throat)

- swelling, inflammation, and redness of tongue

- vascularization of cornea

Clinical signs of deficiency generally appear at intakes of less than 0.5 to 0.6 mg/day. A variety of conditions may produce riboflavin deficiency such as:

- alcoholics are reported to be at increased risk for riboflavin deficiency due to malnutrition, decreased absorption and impaired utilization of the vitamin.

- individuals with an anorexic eating disorder rarely consume adequate riboflavin and may develop a deficiency.

- lactose intolerant individuals may have to refrain from consuming milk or dairy products, reasonably rich sources of riboflavin, and develop a deficiency state.

- hypothyroidism and adrenal insufficiency may impair conversion of riboflavin to the coenzymes FAD and FMN with corresponding decreases in activity.

- physically very active athletes and laborers may have increased riboflavin requirements resulting in a deficiency state, decreasing exercise tolerance, performance or work capacity.

Women at risk of preeclampsia who are riboflavin deficient are reported to be 4-5 times more likely to develop preeclampsia.

Around 25% of independent living people over the age of 65 are reported to consume less than the recommended riboflavin intake. Available evidence indicates that there may be a role for riboflavin in the prevention of age related cataracts in the elderly. Elderly individuals with cataracts also are reported to have among the lowest riboflavin blood levels and nutritional states.

A number of plant and animal derived foods contain significant amounts of riboflavin. Wheat flour and bread are fortified with riboflavin. Reasonably good food sources for riboflavin include fortified cereals, milk, eggs (cooked), almonds, salmon and asparagus.

Sunlight exposure is reported to destroy riboflavin, and up to 50% contained in a clear bottle can be lost after two hours exposure to bright sunlight.

Riboflavin supplements may cause the urine to become bright yellow, a harmless side effect called flavinuria.

IOM has not established a safe, tolerable upper level of intake (UL).

Additional riboflavin information and food sources may be found at:
http://lpi.oregonstate.edu/infocenter/vitamins/riboflavin/riboflavin.html
http://www.nlm.nih.gov/medlineplus (search "riboflavin")
http://www.foodstandards.gov.uk

6.3.6 Vitamin B-3 (Niacin)

Niacin (nicotinic acid/nicotinamide) is a water soluble essential vitamin, also known as vitamin B-3. Both nicotinic acid and nicotinamide, as their respective coenzymes, nicotinamide adenine dinucleotide (NAD) and nicotinamide adenine dinucleotide phosphate (NADP), are required in a number of important enzymatic oxidation/reduction processes. For example, NAD functions in the degradation (breakdown/catabolism) of carbohydrates, fats, protein, and alcohol to produce energy for the body. NADP acts principally in the synthesis of fatty acids and cholesterol. Niacin also is involved in DNA replication and repair as well as cell signaling and differentiation suggesting a possible role in cancer. The amino acid tryptophan is converted in the body to niacin, NAD and NADP. The synthesis of niacin from tryptophan depends on enzymes that require vitamin B-6 (pyridoxine) and vitamin B-2 (riboflavin).

Deficiency of niacin may result in pellagra (from the Italian words pell and agra translated as rough skin) which involves the skin, as well as the digestive and nervous systems producing the four D's: dermatitis, digestive disorders, dementia and death. A dark pigmented rash with thick scaly skin may develop symmetrically in skin areas exposed to sunlight. Digestive problems may include a bright red swollen tongue, diarrhea, and vomiting. Dementia along with apathy, depression, fatigue, disorientation, and memory loss also may occur. Untreated, pellagra may be fatal. Pellagra now is quite uncommon in the United States due in a large measure to supplementation of flour with nicotinic acid since 1939. Now, pellagra occurs most often in chronic alcoholics, and individuals with protein/calorie malnutrition and multiple vitamin deficiency states.

Niacin deficiency usually results from inadequate dietary intake of both niacin and tryptophan. Long term administration of the cancer chemotherapy agent, 5 fluorouricil (5FU) has been reported to cause deficiency symptoms of pellagra. Also, isoniazid treatment of tuberculosis may produce niacin deficiency. Infection with the human immunodeficiency virus (HIV) that causes AIDS is reported to increase tryptophan breakdown in the body and increases the risk of niacin deficiency. Higher levels of niacin intake are associated with decreased progression from HIV infection to AIDs as well as improved survival. Niacin supplements may be considered useful in alcoholism, and with 5FU and isoniazid therapy under a doctor's supervision.

The optimum intake of niacin for health promotion or chronic disease prevention is not known. The DV for niacin is easily obtainable from a varied diet and should prevent niacin deficiency in most people. However, dietary surveys indicate that up to 25% of older people do not consume enough niacin in their diets. Thus, it also may be advisable for older adults and those with poor nutrition to augment their dietary intake with a supplement containing the DV of niacin.

Dietary niacin may be obtained from liver, meat, fish, poultry, whole grain breads and cereals, nuts, and vegetables. Trytophan, a precursor for niacin, is provided by fish as well as animal and other protein sources. In cereal grains like corn and wheat, niacin may be bound to sugar molecules, in the form of glycosides, which significantly decreases its bioavailability.

Research on biochemical and cellular aspects of DNA repair have stimulated interest in the relationship between niacin intake and cancer risk. Increased consumption of niacin along with other antioxidant nutrients is reported to be associated with a decreased incidence of oral (mouth), pharyngeal (throat) and esophageal cancer. Additional studies are needed to confirm these findings and clarify the role of niacin in these cancers.

Pharmocologic doses of nicotinic acid, but not nicotinamide, are known to reduce serum cholesterol. In the Coronary Drug Project, patients who took 3 grams of nicotinic acid daily experienced an average reduction of total blood cholesterol of 10%, triglycerides of 26%, recurrent myocardial infarction of 27%, transient ischemic attacks and stroke of 26%, and total deaths of 10%, over placebo. Other studies have demonstrated that nicotinic acid significantly increases HDL-cholesterol as well. Due to adverse side effects associated with a dose of 3 grams per day, much lower doses of nicotinic acid are now being used successfully in combination with other lipid lowering agents.

Pharmacologic doses of nicotinic acid may produce flushing, skin rashes, itching, headache, nausea and vomiting, and heptotoxicity (liver cell damage) at doses as low as 750 mg per day. Elevated blood levels of uric acid and attacks of gout also may occur in susceptible individuals. Also, taking nicotinic acid with another cholesterol lowering agent such as a "statin drug" may result in rhabdomyolsis, an uncommon form of muscle cell destruction and wasting. levations of blood uric acid and gout with high doses of niacin have been reported as well.

The tolerable safe upper intake level (UL) for niacin is reported to be 35 mg for healthy individuals. This UL is not meant to apply to individuals who are being treated with higher doses of niacin under a doctor's supervision.

Additional niacin information and selected food sources may be found at:
http://lpi.oregonstate.edu/infocenter/vitamins/niacin/niacin.html
http://www.nlm.nih.gov/medlineplus (search "niacin")
http://www.foodstandards.gov.uk

6.3.7 Vitamin B-5 (Pantothenic Acid)

Pantothenic acid is a water soluble essential vitamin, also known as vitamin B-5. It is a component of coenzyme A (coA), an essential factor in a variety of reactions that sustain life. Coenzyme A is required for reactions that:

• generate energy from carbohydrates, fats, and proteins

- are involved in the synthesis of essential fats, cholesterol, and steroid hormones

- produce the neurotransmitter, acetylcholine; the hormone, melatonin; and heme, a component of hemoglobin

- metabolize a number of drugs and toxins in the liver.

Deficiency of pantothenic acid in humans is rare and has been reported to occur chiefly in cases of severe malnutrition. Symptoms of deficiency may include fatigue, headache, insomnia, intestinal disturbances, and numbness of the hands and feet. Anemia may occur due to decreased syntheses of heme and hemoglobin.

Bacteria normally found in the large intestine are capable of making their own pantothenic acid. However, it is not yet known whether humans can absorb this intestinal pantothenic acid made from intestinal bacteria, in significant amounts to prevent deficiency.

Pantothenic acid foods sources include broccoli, egg yolk, chicken, fish, shellfish, milk, yogurt, legumes, mushrooms, avocado, sweet potatoes, and whole grains. Processing of whole grains and freezing and canning of foods may result in a loss of 35-75% of pantothenic acid content.

Pantothenic acid has been demonstrated to accelerate the closure of skin wounds and increase the strength of scar tissue in animals. However, well controlled trials are lacking to demonstrate accelerated wound healing in humans.

Supplements of pantothenic acid commonly contain pantothenol, a more stable alcohol derivative which is converted to pantothenic acid in the body. Calcium and sodium D-pantothenate salts of pantothenic acid also are available as supplements. Pantothenic acid is usually well tolerated in recommended doses, however, diarrhea is reported to occur from doses of 10 to 20 grams per day of calcium D-pantothenate.

The IOM has not established a tolerable safe upper level of intake (UL) for pantothenic acid because of lack of sufficient data to do so.

Evidence is lacking regarding the precise amount of dietary pantothenic acid necessary to promote optimal health or prevent chronic disease. A varied diet is regarded as the best way to ensure adequate daily intake. Older adults and those persons on a poor diet may consider a supplement to ensure adequate intake.

Additional pantothenic acid information and selected food sources may be found at:
http://lpi.oregonstate.edu/infocenter/vitamins/pa/pa.html
http://www.nlm.nih.gov/medlineplus (search "pantothenic acid")
http://www.foodstandards.gov.uk

6.3.8 Vitamin B-6 (Pyridoxine)

Vitamin B-6, pyrodoxine, is a water soluble vitamin that exists principally in three major chemical forms, pyridoxine, pyridoxal and pyridoxamine. It facilitates protein metabolism, red blood cell formation and metabolism, nervous and immune system function, and conversion of tryptophan to niacin. Vitamin B-6 is needed to make hemoglobin and increase the amount of oxygen transported. Deficiency results in a form of anemia similar to iron deficiency anemia.

Through its involvement in protein metabolism and cellular growth, pyrodoxine is important for proper immune function and the health of lymphoid organs (e.g., lymph nodes, spleen, and thymus) that make white blood cells. Deficiency may decease antibody production, and suppress immune response. It also helps to maintain blood sugar levels within a normal range, especially when caloric intake is low, by helping to convert stored carbohydrate or other nutrients to glucose in order to maintain blood sugar levels.

Clinical vitamin B-6 deficiency is uncommonly seen in the United States. However, many older Americans appear to exhibit low blood levels of vitamin B-6 suggesting a marginal vitamin B-6 nutritional status. Outright vitamin B-6 deficiency can occur in individuals with poor quality diets. Clinical symptoms such as dermatitis (skin inflammation) glossitis (sore and inflamed tongue), depression, confusion and convulsions, may occur when vitamin B-6 intake has been very low for an extended period of time. Alcoholics and older adults on poor quality diets are more likely to suffer from inadequate B-6 intake. Alcohol also promotes the destruction and loss of vitamin B-6 from the body. Asthmatics taking theophylline containing medications may need to take a supplement because theophylline decreases body stores of vitamin B-6. Deficiency of vitamin B-6, folic acid, or vitamin B-12 may increase blood level of homocystine, an independent risk factor for heart disease and stroke. Homocystine may damage the arteries, and make it easier for platelets to clump together to form a clot. Lowering homocysteine levels with vitamins may reduce heart attacks and stroke.

Vitamin B-6 is found in a wide variety of foods such as fortified breakfast cereals, fish (e.g., salmon and tuna), meats (e.g., pork and chicken), bananas, beans, peanut butter and many vegetables. Most deficiency states may be corrected by proper dietary intake. When this is not possible, dietary supplements of B-6 may be used.

Isoniazid, used to treat tuberculosis, and L-DOPA used to treat Parkinson's disease, alter the activity of vitamin B-6. Some doctors recommend taking a B-6 supplement providing 100% of the RDA for the vitamin when these drugs are prescribed.

IOM has established safe upper tolerable intake level (UL) for vitamin B-6 of 100 mg per day for adults. The risk of adverse effects is reported to increase as the intake of vitamin B-6 increases above the UL. Motor and sensory neuropathy involving the arms and legs may be related to high intake of vitamin B-6 from supplements. It usually is reversible when supplementation is discontinued.

Additional pyridoxine information and selected food sources may be found at:
http://www.cc.nih.gov/ccc/supplements/vitb6.html
http://www.nlm.nih.gov/medlineplus (search "pyridoxine")
http://www.foodstandards.gov.uk

6.3.9 Vitamin B-9 (Folate/Folic Acid)

Folate and folic acid are two forms of this water soluble B-9 vitamin involved in the production and maintenance of cells, including the manufacture of DNA and RNA (the building blocks of cells) and prevention of changes in DNA that may lead to cancer. Harvard University researchers have reported that individuals with an intake of 400 micrograms per day of folate may cut the risk of colon cancer by more than 50%. Those with a family history of colon cancer had their risk reduced to normal, and women with no family history reduced their risk by around 20%. Folate also is needed to make normal red blood cells and prevent anemia.

Leafy greens and turnip greens, dry beans and peas, fortified cereals and whole grain products and some fruits and vegetables are good sources of folate. In 1998 the Food and Drug Administration (FDA) required the addition of folic acid to enriched breads, cereals, flours, corn meals, pastas, rice and other grain products to reduce the risk of neural tube birth defects and other deficiency syndromes. Fortified foods now have become a major source of folic acid in the American diet.

Deficiency of folate occurs when the need for folate increases, or when dietary folate is inadequate. The need for more folate occurs chiefly in certain conditions such as alcoholism, anemias, kidney and liver diseases, malabsorption syndromes, and malnutrition.

Medications also may interfere with folate utilization, including: anticonvulsants (for epilepsy), metformin (for diabetes), methotrexate (for cancer), sulfasalazine (for intestinal inflammation), and triamterence (for diuresis).

Signs of folate deficiency include diarrhea, loss of appetite, weight loss, weakness, sore tongue, headache, palpitations, irritability, and behavior disorders. Folate supplementation may be useful in such instances as well as cases of anemia (due to folate deficiency), individuals with malabsorption, liver disease, patients receiving kidney dialysis, and those with elevation of homocysteine levels in blood, an independent risk factor for heart disease and stroke.

Additional folate/folic acid information and selected food sources may be found at:
http://www.cc.nih.gov/ccc/supplements/folate.html
http://www.nlm.nih.gov/medlineplus (search "folate")
http://www.foodstandards.gov.uk

6.3.10 Vitamin B-12 (Cobalamin)

Vitamin B-12, helps to maintain healthy nerves and red blood cells, and make DNA. It is bound to protein in food and is released by hydrochloric acid in the stomach during digestion. After release, B-12 combines with a protein, called intrinsic factor in the stomach, needed for absorption.

Most adults receive recommended amounts of vitamin B-12 from their diet. Deficiency usually occurs as a result of inability to absorb B-12 from food, especially in individuals with diets that exclude animal, fish or fortified foods. Also, most individuals who develop a vitamin B-12 deficiency have an underlying stomach disorder (e.g., achlorhydria, or decreased acid production, especially in the elderly), or an intestinal disorder such as celiac disease, sprue, or diarrhea that limits absorption.

Anemia may be the only sign of B-12 deficiency. Fatigue, weakness, nausea, constipation, flatulence (gas), loss of appetite, and weight loss are some of the signs of B-12 deficiency. Inability to maintain balance, confusion, depression, poor memory, and soreness of the mouth or tongue may also occur.

Folic acid can correct the anemia caused by vitamin B-12 deficiency but unfortunately does not correct the underlying B-12 deficiency itself, and permanent nerve damage can occur if the vitamin B-12 deficiency is not treated.

B-12 supplements, have been found to be useful in individuals with pernicious anemia, gastrointestinal disorders and malabsorption, poor diet, vegetarian diets and hearing loss as people age

Increased intake and/or supplements of vitamin B-12 may help protect the hearing of people who work in noisy places. Nearly half the men with tinnitus (annoying ringing and buzzing noise in the ear), as well as measurable loss of hearing due to high decibel workplaces are reported to be deficient in vitamin B-12, and may benefit from increased intake or supplements of this vitamin.

Vitamin B-12, folate, or vitamin B-6 deficiency may decrease blood levels of homocysteine, considered to be an independent risk factor for heart disease and stroke. However, it remains to be determined whether supplementation with vitamin B-12, folic acid, or vitamin B-6 is protective against these disorders.

Adverse effects are unusual even with high intakes of vitamin B-12 from food or supplements.

Adequate vitamin B-12 may be obtained from fortified foods such as breakfast cereals. Adults over 50 years of age should obtain most of their vitamin B-12 from supplements or fortified foods because of the high incidence of impaired absorption in this population

Additional vitamin B-12 information and selected food sources may be found at:
http://www.cc.nih.gov/ccc/supplements/vitb12.html
http://www.nlm.nih.gov/medlineplus (search "vitamin B-12")
http://www.foodstandards.gov.uk

6.4 Major Minerals

The three major minerals, calcium, magnesium and phosphorous are discussed in sections 6.4.1-6.4.3 respectively.

6.4.1 Calcium

Calcium is an essential major mineral for health and the most common one in the body. Around 99% is found in bone and teeth, the remaining 1% is in blood and soft tissues. It plays key roles in:

- blood clotting, acting in conjunction with vitamin K dependent clotting factors involved in the coagulation cascade that stops bleeding.

- cell signaling mediating constriction (vasoconstriction) and relaxation (vasodilation) of blood vessels, nerve impulse transmission, muscle contraction, and the secretion of hormones such as insulin.

- regulation of calcium levels in blood to preserve normal physiological functioning. Parathyroid hormone (PTH) is released to stimulate the conversion of vitamin D to its active form, calcitriol, to increase the absorption of calcium from the intestine. PTH and calcitriol together stimulate the release of calcium from bone by activating bone osteoclasts (bone resorbing cells) and decreasing the excretion of calcium in the urine (by increasing resorption of calcium by the kidneys). When blood calcium is normal, the parathyroid gland stops secreting PTH and the kidneys excrete any excess calcium in the urine, maintaining tight control over concentrations of calcium in the blood and fluid that surrounds cells.

Average dietary intake of calcium in the United States is reported to be well below that recommended by the IOM for male and female adults of:

- 1,000 mg/day for ages 19-50

- 1,200 mg/day 51 years and older

Dairy foods provide around 75% of the calcium in the American diet. While certain plant foods such as broccoli, bok choy, cabbage, mustard and turnip greens contain calcium, it is not as available from these sources as from milk. White beans, tofu, Chinese cabbage, spinach and rhubarb also are considered to be good dietary sources for calcium.

The safe, tolerable upper level for calcium (UL) is 2,500 mg/day for both adult males and females.

Oxalic acid (oxalate) found in significant concentrations in beans (snap), brussel sprouts, carrots, cassava, chives, collards, garlic, lettuce, parsley, purslane, radish, spinach, rhubarb, sweet potato and watercress may inhibit calcium absorption. For oxalic acid content of selected vegetables, see: http://www.nal.usda.gov/fnic/foodcomp/Data/other/oxalic.html

Phytic acid, (phytate) in foods, is a less potent inhibitor of calcium absorption. Yeast has an enzyme, phytase, that breaks down phytic acid in grains during fermentation lowering its content in breads and other fermented foods. However, only concentrated sources of phytate such as wheat bran or dried beans significantly reduce calcium absorption from foods.

Absorption of calcium from food in the intestine is reported to be affected by a number of other factors, namely:

- parathyroid hormone stimulation of the formation of active vitamin D which increases calcium absorption from the intestines.

- adequate amounts of the active form of vitamin D, calcitriol, are needed for satisfactory absorption of calcium

- the body absorbs calcium less efficiently as intake increases. As a result, calcium should be consumed in doses not to exceed 500 mg at any one time.

- dissolution of calcium supplement tablets is a major factor affecting calcium absorption. Tablets should dissolve in 30-40 minutes per U.S.P. standards.

- estrogen increases the production of active vitamin D which in turn increases calcium absorption.

- insoluble fiber found in certain foods such as wheat bran and celery can bind calcium in the intestine and decrease its absorption.

- diarrhea caused by laxative excess can decrease calcium absorption.

- phosphorous and magnesium require vitamin D for absorption and diminish the availability of this vitamin for the absorption of calcium.

- tannins found in tea and coffee also can bind calcium in the intestine and decrease its absorption.

Individuals with a deficiency of calcium in the diet and a low bone density, are at an 80-90% greater risk of having gum disease, the major cause of tooth decay/loss in individuals over 35. Increased calcium intake may reverse this process.

Deficiency of calcium, most often due to inadequate dietary intake, may result in hypocalcemia (low blood calcium levels), osteopenia, and osteoporosis. These disorders are largely preventable by adequate dietary and/or supplemental calcium intake. While supplemental calcium alone usually cannot restore lost bone in individuals with osteoporosis, prevention or treatment may be accomplished by a daily intake of 1,200 mg/day of calcium, 400 IU of vitamin D, and exercise.

Animal and human studies also support a protective role for calcium in preventing intestinal polyps/cancer, particularly in individuals with increased circulating levels of a growth factor, IGF-1. However, further studies are needed before definitive conclusions can be reached regarding the role of calcium in decreasing the risk of colorectal cancer.

The DASH (Dietary Approaches to Stop Hypertension) clinical trials provided evidence that a calcium intake of 1,000-1,200 mg/day also may be helpful in preventing and treating mild to moderate hypertension.

About half of an adult's skeletal mass is accrued during the teenage years. Adult women who consume less than a glass of milk a day during childhood are reported to have more brittle bones and a twofold greater risk of fractures. An 8 ounce glass of milk or a serving of yogurt provides around 300 milligrams of calcium. Comparable amounts of calcium can be obtained from calcium fortified soy milk or cereal, or a glass of orange juice. Milk also is fortified with vitamin D which the body needs to absorb calcium from the intestines. Lactose, milk's major sugar/carbohydrate, also aids in calcium absorption.

In addition research indicates that the importance of calcium extends well beyond bone health. Calcium added to the diet in recommended amounts:

• helps to lower blood pressure in about 1/3 of individuals with hypertension

• improves blood lipid levels by increasing HDL (high density lipoprotein) and lowering LDL (low density lipoprotein) to the extent that may reduce cardiovascular disease by up to 20-30%

• may reduce colon cancer by around 30%

• may play a role in ameliorating symptoms of the premenstrual syndrome, and polycystic ovary syndrome.

Increasing calcium intake in the form of the suggested three glasses of low fat milk per day provides necessary daily calcium intake that may help prevent osteoporosis (which accounts for more than 1.5 million fractures, including 300,000 broken hips each year). Discussion of the pros and cons regarding calcium and milk may be found at:
http://www.hsph.harvard.edu/nutritionsource/calcium.html

One should obtain as much calcium as feasible from foods. However, calcium supplements may be necessary for those who have difficulty doing so. Calcium preparations used as supplements include calcium carbonate, calcium citrate, and others. Calcium carbonate is generally regarded as the most economical. To maximize absorption, calcium carbonate should be taken with meals. The citrate form may be taken between meals. Calcium in a supplement is referred to as elemental calcium. A tablet of 500 mg of calcium carbonate contains only 40% or 200 mg of elemental calcium because 40% is elemental calcium and 60% or 300 mg is the carbonate component.

Additional calcium information and selected food sources may be found at:
http://lpi.oregonstate.edu/infocenter/minerals/calcium/calcium.html
http://ag.arizona.edu/pubs/health/az1042.html
http://www.nlm.nih.gov/medlineplus (search "calcium")
http://www.foodstandards.gov.uk

6.4.2 Magnesium

Magnesium is an essential mineral needed by all cells of the body. Around 50% of the magnesium is inside cells/tissues/organs of the body, and most of the rest is combined with calcium and phosphorous in bone. Only around 1% is in blood. It is needed for hundreds of biochemical reactions in the body involved in maintaining normal muscle and nervous system function, heart rhythm, and bone strength as well as being involved in energy metabolism and protein synthesis.

Magnesium is present in many foods in small amounts. Thus, daily dietary needs cannot easily be met from a single food source. It is necessary to eat a variety of foods including fruits and vegetables as well as whole grains daily to obtain an adequate intake of magnesium. Green vegetables are a good source of magnesium because the chlorophyll molecule contains magnesium in its center. Nuts, seeds and whole grains also are good sources of magnesium. Whole wheat bread has twice the magnesium content of white bread (because the magnesium rich germ and bran are removed to process white flour). Water also can provide magnesium, according to the water supply, with hard water containing more magnesium than soft water.

Many Americans consume less than optimal magnesium in their diets, however, frank deficiency is uncommon in adults. Conditions in which there is an excessive loss in urine, or limitation absorption, or a chronically low intake account for most of the cases of magnesium deficiency in the United States. Poorly controlled diabetes, alcohol, diuretics, some antibiotics, and some medicine used to treat cancer such as cisplatin, may increase loss of magnesium in urine, and produce deficiency. Malabsorption disorders such as sprue, celiac disease, excessive vomiting, and diarrhea may cause a loss and/or limit absorption of magnesium with resultant deficiencies. Chronically low intake, particularly in the elderly on an inadequate diet may also result in magnesium deficiency.

Healthy adults who consume a varied diet generally do not need to take a magnesium supplement. However, when a health problem or condition causes excessive loss or limits absorption, magnesium supplementation may be indicated.

Increased magnesium intake is associated with a lower risk of hypertension. The Joint National Committee on Prevention, Detection, Evaluation, and Treatment of High Blood Pressure recommends an adequate magnesium intake as a positive lifestyle modification for preventing and managing high blood pressure and its implications. Low body stores of magnesium increase the risk of abnormal heart rhythms that may increase the risk of complications following a heart attack. And dietary surveys suggest that a higher magnesium intake is associated with a lower risk of stroke. In patients with hypertension, consideration should be given to increasing magnesium intake through a supplement under a doctor's supervision.

Magnesium deficiency also is regarded as a risk factor for postmenopausal osteoporosis. It affects calcium metabolism, and supplementation may improve bone mineral density.

Magnesium is reported to influence the release and activity of insulin. Elevated blood glucose levels increase the loss of magnesium in urine which in turn lowers blood levels of magnesium. And, low blood levels of magnesium are associated with poorly controlled types I and II diabetes. Magnesium supplementation, in cases in which blood levels of magnesium are found to be low, may help to improve control of diabetes.

IOM has established a safe upper intake level (UL) for magnesium at 350 mg daily. As intake increases above the UL, the risk of adverse effects increases. Magnesium supplements in patients using laxatives can produce diarrhea. Also, the elderly are at risk of magnesium toxicity because kidney function declines with age, and such individuals are more likely to take magnesium containing laxatives and antacids. Mental status changes, nausea, diarrhea, loss of appetite, muscle weakness, difficulty breathing, low blood pressure and irregular heart beat are common to both magnesium excess and magnesium deficiency.

Additional magnesium information and selected food sources are available at:
http://www.cc.nih.gov/ccc/supplements/magn.html
http://www.nlm.nih.gov/medlineplus (search "magnesium")
http://www.foodstandards.gov.uk

6.4.3 Phosphorous

Phosphorous is an essential mineral that is required by all cells in the body for normal function and health. It exists principally as phosphate (PO4) in the body and approximately 85% is found in bone.

Phosphorous is a major component of:

- a calcium phosphate salt called hydroxyappetite giving bone its strength

- cell membrane phospholipids and structure/function

- phosphorylated compounds used for energy production and storage, such as adenosine triphosphate or ATP

- nucleic acids, DNA and RNA, responsible for the storage and transmission of genetic information

- enzymes, hormones, and cell signaling molecules dependent on phosphorylation for activation

- the buffering system that helps maintain normal acid base balance

- a phosphorous containing molecule that binds to hemoglobin in red cells and aids oxygen delivery to the tissues of the body

Under normal circumstances, dietary phosphorous is readily absorbed from the small intestine and any excess absorbed is excreted by the kidneys in the urine. Blood and cellular phosphorous and calcium are regulated by vitamin D and parathyroid hormone.

A diet high in fructose is reported to increase the urinary loss of phosphorous and may produce a negative phosphorous balance (when loss becomes larger than intake). Low magnesium intake tends to increase this loss of phosphorous. Increased consumption of food products containing high fructose corn syrup and decreased magnesium intake over most of the last part of this century has raised concerns in this regard.

Some research indicates that high dietary phosphorous intake may be detrimental to bone health. Much of the high intake of phosphorous in the diet can be attributed to phosphoric acid in soft drinks and phosphate additives in a number of commercially prepared foods. However, convincing evidence that high dietary intake of phosphorous alone adversely affects bone mineral density in humans is lacking at this time. Nevertheless, it should be borne in mind that substitution of phosphate containing soft drinks and snack foods for milk and other calcium containing foods may represent a serious risk for bone health.

Inadequate intake of phosphorous may result in low serum phosphate levels, a condition referred to as hypophospatemia. This condition may include anemia, bone pain, difficulty in walking, loss of appetite, muscle weakness, numbness and tingling of the extremities, osteomalacia (in adults), rickets (in children), susceptibility to infection, and death. However, since phosphorous is so widespread and readily available from food, phosphorous deficiency usually occurs only in those suffering from severe malnutrition.

Individuals at risk of hypophosphatemia include alcoholics, diabetics with ketoacidosis, those who are severely malnourished or starving, and anorectic patients on feeding regimens very low in phosphorous and high in calories.

Almonds, dairy products, lentils, fish and meat are good sources of phosphorous. Polyphosphate food additives and some soft drinks may serve as a good source of phosphorous as well. Phosphorous in all plant seeds (beans, peas, cereals and nuts) is contained in a tightly bound storage form of phosphate called phytic acid or phytate, and is only around 50% available to humans because of the lack of necessary enzymes, the phytases, to liberate phosphorous. Since yeast has phytases, whole grains in leavened breads, or cereals have more phosphorous that is available to humans. Phosphate supplements used for the treatment of hypophosphatemia require medical supervision because of potential toxicity. The IOM has established a safe, tolerable upper intake level

(UL) of 4 grams per day in adults, 3 grams/day in individuals 70 years or older. Multivitamin/mineral supplements contain less than 15% of the current RDA/DV for phosphorous and thus are not useful as a supplement for deficiency. However, a varied diet of good food sources for phosphorous should easily provide adequate phosphorous intake for most individuals.

Absorption of dietary phosphorous is decreased by aluminum containing antacids due to the formation of aluminum phosphate which is not absorbed.

Additional phosphorous information and selected food sources may be found at:
http://lpi.oregeonstate.edu/infocenter/minerals/phosphorus/phosphorus.html
http://www.nlm.nih.gov/medlineplus (search "phosphorous")
http://www.foodstandards.gov.uk

6.5 Mineral Electrolytes

The three essential mineral electrolytes, sodium, chloride and potassium are discussed in sections 6.5.1-6.5.2 respectively.

6.5.1 Sodium/Chloride (Salt)

Sodium and chloride are essential for life. Sodium and chloride electrolyte concentrations are so important that the body employs multiple mechanisms working in concert to control their levels in the body. They are the extracellular fluid electrolytes (including blood plasma), that play a critical role in many life sustaining processes. They contribute to the maintenance of charge and concentration differences across cell membranes. Sodium is the principal positively charged ion (cation) in extracellular (outside cells) fluid whereas potassium concentrations are about 30 times higher inside, compared with outside cells. These concentration differences across cell membranes create an electrochemical gradient known as the membrane potential that is maintained by sodium/potassium ATP pumps. Approximately 20-40% of the resting energy expenditure of a typical adult is used by these pumps in order to maintain sodium/potassium concentration gradients needed to sustain life. Precise control of cell membrane potential is critical for cardiac function, muscle contraction, and nerve impulse transmission.

Absorption of chloride and other substances such as amino acids, glucose, and water are dependent on the uptake of sodium from the small intestine. Resorption of these nutrients after they have been filtered from the blood by the kidneys is accomplished by similar mechanisms involving sodium. On the other hand, chloride becomes hydrochloric acid (HCl) in gastric juice that assists in the digestion and absorption of other nutrients.

A number of physiological mechanisms that regulate blood volume and blood pressure adjust the body's sodium content. Generally sodium retention in the body results in water retention and sodium loss is followed by water loss. This is accomplished principally by two mechanisms, namely the:

- renin angiotension—aldosterone system, and

- anti-diuretic hormone.

Both help regulate extracellular fluid, blood volume and blood pressure within a healthy range.

Sodium/chloride (salt) deficiency is defined as a serum sodium concentration of less than 136 (millimols/liter). Generally, deficiency does not occur as a result of inadequate dietary intake or even as a result of very low salt diets. However, deficiency may result from increased loss of sodium and chloride from severe or prolonged vomiting or diarrhea, excessive or persistent sweating, use of some diuretics, and less commonly from some forms of kidney disease. Symptoms of salt deficiency may include headache, fatigue, fainting, muscle cramps, nausea, vomiting, low blood pressure, and disorientation. Rapidly developing salt deficiency may result in edema (swelling) of the brain, seizures, brain damage, and death.

The IOM has established Minimum Daily Requirements (MDRs) at 500 mg/day for sodium and 250 mg/day for chloride for both men and women. No allowance is provided for large, prolonged losses from the skin through sweat. And, it should be noted that these minimal requirements are well below the average dietary intakes of most adults.

Epidemiologic studies indicate that high intakes of salted, smoked and pickled foods increase the risk of gastric cancer. While such foods are high in salt, they may also contain nitrosamines, known carcinogens for causing gastric cancer.

Populations that consume such foods also tend to have low intakes of fruits and vegetables that also may contribute to the risk of gastric cancer. Salt alone, however, does not appear to act as a carcinogen for gastric cancer.

Increased salt intake has been reported to increase urinary excretion of calcium and is associated with biochemical markers of bone resorption and decreased bone mineral density (BMD) in postmenopausal women. Also each 2.3 grams increment of sodium (5.8 grams of salt) excreted by the kidneys has been found to draw 20-40 milligrams of calcium into the urine. Further studies are needed to determine whether decreasing salt intake has clinically significant effects on BMD and fractures in individuals at risk for osteoporosis.

A sodium intake averaging around 5 grams/day (12 grams of salt) may increase the risk of developing symptomatic kidney stones due to increased calcium excretion. In contrast, a diet low in sodium and animal protein may decrease stone recurrence.

Dietary salt restriction has been found to lower blood pressure significantly in 30-60% of hypertensive and 25-50% of normotensive individuals, suggesting that a subset of people are sensitive to the effects of dietary salt on blood pressure. Such salt sensitivity appears to occur more often in obese and insulin resistant people, as well as black, elderly, and female hypertensive individuals. In such salt sensitive patients, lowering salt intake results in a clinically significant decrease in blood pressure.

The DASH (Dietary Approaches to Stop Hypertension) trial demonstrated that a diet with a low salt/high calcium and potassium intake (emphasizing fruits, vegetables, grains, poultry, fish, nuts and low fat dairy products), significantly lowers blood pressure in hypertensive individuals. The vast majority (75%) of sodium and chloride in the diet is obtained from salt added during food processing or manufacturing, rather than salt added during cooking or at the lunch or dinner table. Diets that emphasize unprocessed foods such as fruits, vegetables, and legumes provide the lowest salt intake. As a result the National High Blood Pressure Education Program (NHBPEP) and the National Heart, Lung, and Blood Institute (NHLBI) recommend consuming no more than 6 grams/day of salt (equivalent to around 2.4 grams/day of sodium) which is around 4 grams/day less than the national average. US Dietary Guidelines recommend no more than 5.8 grams/day of salt per day.

Other studies have shown that high salt intake is significantly correlated with left ventricular hypertropy, an abnormal thickening of the left ventricle heart muscle, which is associated with increased mortality from cardiovascular disease. High intakes of salt also may lead to an increase in extracellular fluid. Ingestion of large amounts of salt may lead to nausea, vomiting, diarrhea, abdominal cramps, and abnormally high plasma sodium concentrations with edema (swelling), hypertension, rapid heart rate, difficult in breathing, heart failure, convulsions and death.

Among drugs, diuretics are the chief cause of drug induced sodium deficiency. Other drugs also may play a role.

Additional sodium/salt information and selected food sources are available at:
http://lpi.oregeonstate.edu/infocenter/minerals/sodium/sodium.html
http://www.nlm.nih.gov/medlineplus (search "sodium")
http://www.foodstandards.gov.uk

6.5.2 Potassium

Potassium is an essential mineral electrolyte and the principal positively charged ion (cation) in the fluid inside cells (around 30 times higher inside compared with outside cells). In contrast, sodium concentrations are more than 10 times lower inside compared with outside cells. These concentration gradients create an electrochemical membrane potential that is maintained by an ion pumps, the sodium/potassium ATPase pumps. Daily activity of these pumping systems accounts for 20-40% of the resting energy expenditure in an average adult. Narrow control of the cell membrane potential is important for proper heart function, muscle contraction, and nerve impulse transmission.

Potassium serves as a cofactor for a limited number of key enzyme systems. For example, potassium is required for the:

- sodium/potassium ATPase pump system for regulation of cell membrane potential

- pyruvate kinase system involved in carbohydrate metabolism

- other key enzyme systems as well.

Deficiency of potassium results in low potassium concentrations in blood and cells, and this is referred to as hypokalemia. This disorder may include muscular weakness and cramps, fatigue, intestinal paralysis, and abnormal heart rhythms and abdominal pain. Generally, low dietary intakes of potassium do not result in hypokalemia, however, insufficient dietary intake of potassium may increase the risk of certain chronic diseases such as hypertension, kidney stones, osteopenia/osteoporosis, and stroke. Potassium deficiency is uncommon except in certain medical conditions. For example, some heart and high blood pressure medications such as diuretics increase urination and potassium loss and may lead to a deficiency. Other conditions that may increase the risk of insufficient dietary intake of potassium, include alcoholism and malnutrition, congestive heart failure, eating disorders such as anorexia nervosa, laxative over use/abuse, magnesium depletion, and malabsorption syndromes and diarrhea.

A Recommended Daily Allowance (RDA) for potassium has not been established by the IOM. However, it estimates the Minimum Daily Requirement (MDR) for potassium to be 2 grams/day for adult males and females. Daily Value is set at 4 grams/day for males and females which most people can obtain by eating a balanced diet.

Epidemiological studies indicate that increased intake of potassium in the diet is associated with a decreased risk of stroke. Studies also have provided evidence for a positive association between dietary potassium intake and bone mineral density, especially in the elderly. Potassium rich foods contain precursors to bicarbonate ions (alkali) which serve to buffer acids in the body and preserve calcium in bones. This evidence suggests that high dietary potassium intake from fruits and vegetables and other foods may be protective against osteopenia (decreased mineralization of bone) and osteoporosis (decreased bone matrix). Increased dietary intake of potassium and alkali from food also may decrease the formation of calcium containing kidney stones.

Individuals with increased dietary potassium intake tend to have significantly lower blood pressure. The DASH (Dietary Approaches to Stop Hypertension) trials provided evidence to support the beneficial effect of a potassium rich diet on blood pressure. Also, increasing dietary calcium intake by 800 mg/day was found to lower blood pressure even further in these trials.

A potassium rich diet (fruits, vegetables and legumes) may also enable a significant number of mild to moderate hypertensive patients to reduce, or even discontinue, their antihypertensive medications(s). Potassium supplements also are reported to reduce blood pressure significantly in hypertensive patients, particularly in those individuals with high salt intakes.

Fruits and vegetables are among the richest sources of potassium. Bananas, juices (prune, tomato, and orange), raisin bran cereal, and spinach are considered to be good dietary potassium food sources. Individuals who eat significant amounts of fruits and vegetables usually have a reasonably high potassium intake of 4 grams or more/day and a decreased risk of hypertension, kidney stones, osteopenia, osteoporosis and stroke.

Foods that provide increased potassium intake include:

Food (calories)	Milligrams Potassium
one baked potato with skin (210)	900
one cup prune juice (180)	700
five dried peach halves (150)	650
one baked potato with no skin (150)	640
one cup low fat yogurt (130)	500
one half cup cooked Swiss chard (20)	480
ten dried apricot halves (80)	480
one cup orange juice from concentrate (110)	470
one banana (100)	450
one half cup cooked squash (60)	450
one half cup spinach (20)	420
three quarter cup tomato juice (30)	400

Increased potassium intake from foods generally may be considered reasonably safe. However, potassium supplements should only be taken under a doctor's supervision because of potential serious side effects such as hyperkalemia, cardiac arrythmias, and intestinal ulceration and bleeding.

Additional potassium information and selected food sources are available at:
http://lpi.oregeonstate.edu/infocenter/minerals/potassium/potassium.html
http://www.mayoclinic.com
http://www.nlm.nih.gov/medlineplus (search "potassium")
http://www.foodstandards.gov.uk

6.6 Trace Minerals

The 10 essential trace minerals are discussed in sections 6.6.1-6.6.10 respectively.

6.6.1 Chromium

Chromium is an essential trace mineral that exists in two common forms, trivalent and hexavalent. Trivalent chromium is the principal form in foods used by the body and the subject of discussion.

Hexavalent chromium, on the other hand, is used for industrial/purposes only. Exposure to hexavalent chromium dust is associated with an increased incidence of lung cancer and skin inflammation. It will not be considered further.

Ingested chromium from foods is converted to a biologically active form, the precise structure of which is not known at this time. This biologically active form participates in glucose metabolism enhancing the effects of insulin in transporting glucose into the cells via a low molecular weight chromium binding substance referred to as LMWCr.

Absorption of chromium into the body may be enhanced when given at the same time as vitamin C. Once absorbed, chromium competes for one of the biding sites on the iron transport protein, transferrin, and may decrease transferrin saturation with iron. Diets high in simple sugars increase urinary chromium excretion. The body's need for chromium may be increased by exercise.

Presently, research regarding chromium deficiency is limited by the lack of sensitive and accurate means for determining the chromium nutritional status of individuals. Chromium deficiency may occur in patients on long term intravenous feeding (e.g. total parenteral nutrition) who do not receive supplemental chromium. Such deficiency may be characterized by evidence of abnormal glucose utilization and increased insulin requirements that usually respond to chromium supplementation. Because of this, it has been suggested that chromium deficiency may be a contributing factor in the development of type 2 (non-insulin-dependent) diabetes mellitus.

Chromium supplementation is reported to improve glucose utilization and blood lipid profiles in individuals with impaired glucose tolerance in doses of 200 mcg/day. Impaired glucose tolerance may lead to type 2 diabetes in around 25-30% of cases. Inconsistent results from study to study may mean that individuals with chromium deficiency are the ones experiencing the beneficial effects from chromium supplements.

In patients with type 2 diabetes mellitus, chromium supplementation is reported to reduce blood sugar and insulin levels as well as glycosated hemoglobin, a measure of control of blood sugar levels over time. While further studies are needed to clarify the dose, efficacy, safety, and role of chromium supplements in persons with impaired glucose tolerance and/or type 2 diabetes, chromium supplementation may be considered in diabetics under the supervision of a doctor.

Health claims that chromium supplementation promotes weight loss, increases body muscle mass, and/or decreases body fat do not appear to be supported by available evidence. In fact, the US Federal Trade Commission (FTC) has ruled that there is no basis for such claims in humans.

Chromium content in foods appears to be quite variable and has been measured accurately in only a small number of foods. Processed meats, whole grain products, bran cereal, green beans, broccoli, grape and orange juice, potatoes, English muffins, apples with the peel and some spices appear to be reasonably good sources for dietary chromium.

The IOM has not set a safe, tolerable upper limit of intake (UL) for adults for chromium due to the fact that necessary information upon which to make such a judgement is limited.

Current concerns about chromium safety center chiefly around the piccolinate form. Kidney failure has been reported after a six-week course of 600 mcg of chromium piccolinate. Both kidney failure and impaired liver function has been reported after the use of 1,200 to 2,400 mcg/day of chromium piccolinate following treatment for 4-5 months. Therefore, use of chromium piccolinate supplements is not recommended.

Calcium carbonate and magnesium hydroxide containing antacids may decrease chromium absorption. Aspirin and indomethecin may increase chromium absorption.

Chromium supplements are available in several forms ranging in content from 50 to 200 mcg of elemental chromium. Multiple vitamin/mineral preparations usually contain 30 mcg or 100% of the daily value.

Additional chromium information and selected food sources may be found at: http://lpi.oregeonstate.edu/infocenter/minerals/chromium/chromium.html
http://www.allachlive.com/chromium.htm
http://www.nlm.nih.gov/medlineplus (search "chromium")
http://www.foodstandards.gov.uk

6.6.2 Cobalt

Cobalt is an essential trace mineral. It is found principally in the cobalt containing vitamin B-12 (cobalamin), a mainly animal sourced vitamin. The adult body contains about 10 milligrams of cobalt.

Principal functions of cobalt include those of:

- vitamin B-12 production and action

- production, function, and maintenance of red blood cells

- keeping the antioxidant glutathione biologically active as part of several enzyme systems involved in carbohydrate metabolism

- maintaining a healthy brain and nervous system

- metabolizing protein and fatty acids vital to nerve health

- metabolism of folic acid.

Food sources for cobalt include clams, beef (muscle meats), dairy products, seafood, kidney, liver and other foods of animal origin.

Cobalt is absorbed from the upper part of the small intestine (jejunum) via a path shared by iron. Under normal circumstances, cobalt itself generally is not well absorbed and mostly passes through the intestines into the feces, unabsorbed. Absorption may be improved by gastric juice and vitamins B-2 (riboflavin), B-3 (niacin) and manganese. Calcium plays a role in releasing cobalt containing vitamin B-12 from protein for absorption. Cobalt is stored in the liver, pancreas, and spleen as vitamin B-12 as well as in red blood cells and plasma. The body protects its supply of cobalt containing vitamin B-12, and deficiency requires years to develop.

Plants do not manufacture vitamin B-12 so vegetarians can be at risk of cobalt/vitamin B-12 deficiency. Cobalt deficiency is characterized principally as a B-12 deficiency. Symptoms/signs include those of pernicious anemia and nervous system damage.

In megadoses of 20-30 milligrams/day, cobalt may produce polycythemia and an enlargement of the heart, leading to congestive heart failure, and thyroid gland enlargement. Inorganic cobalt, used to stabilize beer, can be toxic at high intakes and may result in an enlarged thyroid and polycythemia (too many red cells due to an overproduction of the hormone erythropoietin). Cobalt plus alcohol may synergize to produce cardiac problems (cardiomyopauthy and congestive heart failure) principally in heavy beer drinkers.

Additional cobalt information and selected food sources are available at:
http://www.mdadvice.com/library/vita/vitamin19.html
http://www.foodstandards.gov.uk

6.6.3 Copper

Copper is an essential trace mineral with which the body forms hemoglobin and red blood cells, and keeps the immune system, bone development, connective tissue, blood vessels, and the nervous system healthy. It acts as a catalyst to store and release iron to form hemoglobin.

Copper is found in moderate levels in fish, meat, poultry, fruits (such as mangos, pears, pineapples, and papaya), vegetables (asparagus, bean sprouts, broccoli, spinach, and tomatoes), grains (whole grains bread, cereals), olives, potatoes, pumpkin, melba toast, parsnips, winter squash, ketchup, and canned soups. The concentration of copper in foods depends on geographical sources, plant or animal species, and soil conditions, among other factors.

Deficiency of copper is uncommon in the United States. It may be characterized by anemia, growth retardation, defective keratinization and pigmentation of hair, hypothermia, degenerative changes in the aorta, mental deterioration, and scurvy like changes in bone.

Toxicity may be manifested as abdominal pain, nausea and vomiting, diarrhea, hepatitis, cirrhosis, tremor, mental deterioration, hemolytic anemia, kidney dysfunction (Fanconi-like syndrome), and even death.

Dietary copper intake may need to be reduced when certain medical conditions are present that affect how the body absorbs, uses, or excretes copper. These may include:

1. bile flow obstruction (bile is the principal way the body excretes copper)

2. excessive copper supplements (excessive copper intake unsupervised by a medical doctor)

3. hemodialysis (when dialysis solutions are contaminated with excessive copper)

4. Wilson's disease (genetic disorder resulting in retention of copper by the body)

Foods high in copper content need to be avoided, and foods with a moderate copper content need to be restricted in such instances.

Additional copper information and selected food sources may be found at:
http://lpi.oregeonstate.edu/infocenter/minerals/copper/copper.html
http://www.nlm.nih.gov/medlineplus (search "copper")
http://wwwstandards.food.gov.uk

6.6.4 Fluorine

Fluorine is a trace element that occurs in the body, food and water as the negatively charged ion (anion). It is generally not considered an essential mineral since it is not required for growth or to sustain life. However, fluorine's role in the prevention of tooth decay (dental caries) has been established and this serves as an important basis upon which to consider fluorine an essential element for humans.

Fluoride is absorbed from the stomach and small intestine, rapidly enters bone and developing teeth and does not accumulate in soft tissue. Bone normally contains principally calcium and phosphate as hydroxyapatite crystals. Fluoride displaces the hydroxyl ion in hydroxyapatite forming fluoroapatite that hardens tooth enamel and stabilizes bone mineral density. Calcium supplements, as well as calcium and aluminum antacids, decrease the absorption of fluoride. Both calcium and magnesium may form insoluble complexes with fluoride and significantly decrease fluoride absorption. Deficiency of fluoride intake in the diet increases tooth decay for individuals of all ages. In contrast, tooth decay has been found to be much lower in communities with optimal water fluoride concentrations.

The IOM has not established a RDA for fluoride because of inadequate data upon which to do so. Rather, Adequate Intake (AI) levels have been set at 0.05 milligrams/kilogram of body weight, the level shown to reduce the occurrence of tooth decay (dental caries) most effectively without causing the undesirable side effect of tooth enamel mottling known as dental fluorosis. On this basis, an adult AI has been established at 4 mg/day for males and 3 mg/day for females.

Cavity causing bacteria (cariogenic) found in dental plaque metabolize certain sugars into organic acids that dissolve tooth enamel resulting in tooth decay. By adding fluoride to community water supplies, caries are reduced by up to 60%. When enamel is partially demineralized by these organic acids, fluoride may enhance the remineralization through interactions with calcium and phosphate, and the remineralized enamel becomes more resistant to further demineralization. Fluoride also has been found to inhibit bacterial enzymes in plaque reducing organic acid production and consequent destruction of enamel.

Fluoridated drinking water is the major source of dietary fluoride in the US diet. When drinking water is adjusted to between 0.7 to 1.2 milligrams of fluoride per liter, this has been found to decrease the incidence of dental caries (tooth decay) while minimizing dental fluorosis (mottling or discoloration of the teeth). Most (over 60%) of the US population now consumes sufficient fluoride for the prevention of dental caries, having an average adult fluoride intake of 1.5 to 3.0 mg/day. In this regard, it should be recognized that water softeners do not remove fluoride whereas reverse osmosis units and some water filters (except the Brita type) may remove significant amounts of fluoride from drinking water.

Most commonly consumed foods are low in fluoride content, containing less than 0.05 mg/100 grams. On the other hand, tea (which concentrates fluoride in its leaves), canned sardines (with bones), fish (without bones), hot dogs, and chicken may contribute 0.3 to 0.6 mg of the daily intake of fluoride, and are considered to be good food sources. Fluoridated tooth pastes also add significantly to the daily intake of fluoride.

Extensive scientific research has revealed no significant evidence for any increased risk of chronic diseases such as cancer, heart, kidney or liver disorders due to fluoride intake from food, fluoridated water or toothpaste. However, the risk of mild to moderate fluorosis (discoloration of the teeth) may increase significantly as intake of fluoride increases over 2-3 times recommended intakes for children.

Skeletal fluorosis from excessive intake of fluoride over long periods of time may also occur in adults. This condition is characterized by increased bone mass detected by x-ray along with joint pain and stiffness. Crippling skeletal fluorosis resulting in calcification of ligaments, immobility, muscle wasting and neurological problems related to spinal cord compression may occur when fluoride intake exceeds 10-25 mg/day for years.

Additional fluoride information and selected food sources may be found at:
http://lpi.oregonstate.edu/infocenter/minerals/fluoride/fluoride.html
http://www.nlm.nih.gov/medlineplus (search "fluoride")
http://www.foodstandards.gov.uk

6.6.5 Iodine

Iodine is a nonmetallic essential trace element. It is required by humans for the synthesis of the thyroid hormones, thyroxine (T-4) and triiodothyronine (T-3), and normal thyroid function. Thyroid hormones regulate a number of physiologic processes including growth, development, metabolism and reproduction.

Secretion of thyrotropin releasing hormone (TRH) by the hypothalamus results in the release of thyroid stimulating hormone (TSH) by the pituitary gland which turns on iodine trapping, thyroid hormone synthesis of T-4 and T-3 and their release by the thyroid gland. Normal circulating T-4 in the blood limits increases in TSH. Iodine deficiency results in inadequate production of T-4 by the thyroid gland and a corresponding increase in the output of TSH by the pituitary gland. Chronically elevated TSH levels in blood lead to enlargement of the thyroid gland referred to as a goiter.

Iodine deficiency disorders (IDD) are regarded as among the most preventable in the world. The World Health Organization estimates that around 750 million people around the world suffer from IDD, and some 50 million from related brain damage. Such deficiency states have adverse effects at all stages of development but are most damaging to the developing brain (during prenatal development, in newborns, infants, children and adolescents).

Thyroid enlargement (goiter) is one of the earliest and most visible signs of iodine deficiency in adults. IDD also may produce growth and development abnormalities, hypothyroidism and mental retardation.

Vitamin A, iron, and selenium deficiencies may worsen iodine deficiencies. For example, selenium dependent enzymes (iodothyronine deiodenases) are required for the conversion of thyroxine to the biologically active thyroid hormone, T-3. Also certain foods (those containing compounds called goitrogens) interfere with iodine utilization or thyroid hormone production. These include foods such as casava, cabbage, broccoli, cauliflower, and brussels sprouts. Soybean isoflavones, daidzein and genistein, also inhibit thyroid hormone synthesis. However, goitogens usually are of little clinical significance unless consumed regularly in large amounts, or there already is some degree of iodine deficiency present. Vegetarian diets that exclude iodized salt and fish usually contain little iodine and may enhance goitrogen significance in the diet.

Dairy products are good sources because iodine is added to animal feed, and seafood is rich in content because marine animals concentrate iodine from sea water. Processed foods may contain higher levels because of the addition of iodized salt or food additives such as potassium and calcium iodates. Iodized salt, cod, shrimp, cow's milk, boiled eggs, navy beans, baked potato with peel, baked turkey breast, and seaweed are considered to be good sources of iodine.

Potassium iodide is available as a supplement, typically as part of a multivitamin/mineral product that usually contains 100% of the Daily Value. Iodine makes up around ¾ of the total weight of potassium iodide. Iodized salt contains around 77 mcg of iodine per gram of salt. Iodine toxicity from dietary intake or multivitamin/mineral supplements is uncommon. Individuals who are allergic should refrain from consuming foods high in iodine content or taking iodine supplements, unless done under a doctor's supervision.

In iodine deficient individuals, 150-200 mcg/day of supplemental iodine has been found to increase the incidence of iodine induced hyperthyroidism (IHH), mainly in older people and those with multinodular goiter. In iodine sufficient individuals supplemental iodine intake may be associated with elevated levels of the thyroid stimulating hormone (TSH), hypothyroidism and goiter. Increased iodine intake may also be associated with an increased incidence of thyroid papillary cancer. The safe, tolerable upper level (UL) for iodine is set at 1,100 mcg/day (1.1 milligrams/day) for male and female adults.

Prescription drugs such as amiodarone, an antiarrhythmic agent, contains iodine that may affect thyroid function. Pharmacologic doses of potassium iodide may decrease the anticoagulant (blood thinning) action of warfarin.

Additional iodine information and selected food sources are available at:
http://lpi.oregonstate.edu/infocenter/minerals/iodine/iodine.html
http://www.nlm.nih.gov/medlineplus (search "iodine")
http://www.foodstandards.gov.uk

6.6.6 Iron

Iron is an essential mineral. Around 65% of iron is found in the red blood cells that carry oxygen to the tissues. Much lesser amounts are in myoglobin, the protein that helps supply oxygen to muscle. Smaller amounts can be found in enzymes that assist a variety of essential biochemical reactions in cells. Additional iron is located in body tissues and organ stores that can be mobilized when dietary intake is insufficient. The body usually maintains normal iron content by regulating the amount of iron absorbed from food.

Dietary iron exists in two principal chemical forms, namely, heme and nonheme. Heme iron is found in food sources such as fish, beef and poultry. Nonheme iron is found in plant foods such as lentils and beans.

Around 10-20% of the iron in the diet generally is absorbed. However, absorption may be influenced by body iron stores, type of iron in the diet, and other factors. The amount of iron stored in the body is the chief factor that regulates iron absorption, being greatest when body iron stores are low and decreasing when body iron stores are high, in order to protect against iron overload.

Absorption of heme iron is regarded as very efficient and not significantly affected by the composition of the diet. On the other hand, only around 2% to 7% of nonheme iron in beans, maize, rice and wheat is absorbed when consumed as single foods. However, meat proteins and vitamin C, as well as other dietary factors, can improve the absorption of nonheme iron. Diets that include 5 to 9 servings of fruits and vegetables provide sufficient vitamin C to boost nonheme iron absorption to desired levels.

Certain dietary factors such as calcium, polyphenols and tannins found in tea, and phytates in plant foods such as vegetables/grains/soybeans/rice, may decrease absorption of nonheme iron. Nevertheless, most individuals are able to maintain normal body iron stores when the diet consists of a variety of food sources.

While vegetarians often have iron intakes that are similar to nonvegetarians, less of the iron is absorbed from a vegetarian diet. This is due to the fact that iron from plant foods is in the form of nonheme iron that is not as well absorbed as the heme iron found in meat and fish. The amount of nonheme iron that is absorbed is increased by vitamin C and decreased by phytates (found in dried beans, rice and grains, calcium, tea and coffee). This lower absorption of iron from a vegetarian diet can lead to lower levels of ferritin in the blood. Blood ferritin is an indicator of iron stores, so low ferritin levels indicate that little iron is stored for use when need is greater or intake is less. Based on the lower absorption of iron from a plant based diet, IOM recommends that adult vegetarians obtain 1.8 times more iron than nonvegetarians from their diet.

Iron deficiency is considered one of the most common nutritional disorders in the world by the World Health Organization. It exists when blood and storage levels of iron are low, and the blood hemoglobin level falls below normal due to a low dietary intake, inadequate intestinal absorption, excessive blood loss, or increased needs. Signs of iron deficiency anemia include feelings of tiredness and weakness, decreased concentration and cognition, decreased performance, difficulty in maintaining body temperature, and decreased immune function/resistance to infection.

Iron supplementation is indicated when iron deficiency is diagnosed, and diet alone cannot restore body iron content to normal levels in a reasonable period of time. Supplements come in two forms, ferrous and ferric, with the ferrous form being preferred because it is better absorbed. Iron supplements may interfere with zinc uptake.

Meat, fish, and poultry are good sources of heme iron, beans of nonheme iron. In addition, many foods are fortified with iron. It is important for anyone considering taking an iron supplement to first evaluate the amount natural and fortified dietary heme and nonheme iron that are being consumed to avoid excessive intake.

Iron has a moderate to high potential for toxicity because very little iron is excreted from the body and iron can accumulate in tissues and organs when normal storage sites are full. The IOM has establised a safe upper intake level (UL) of 45 mg per day for adults 19 years of age and older.

Additional trace mineral iron information and selected food sources are available at:
http://www.cc.nih.gov/ccc/supplements/iron.html

http://www.nlm.nih.gov/medlineplus (search "trace mineral iron")
http://www.foodstandards.gov.uk

6.6.7 Manganese

Manganese is an essential antioxidant trace mineral needed for normal growth and health. It aids in the metabolism of fats, carbohydrates and proteins as a part of several enzyme systems in the body. Manganese also appears to be important for normal brain function.

Manganese is found in whole grains, cereal products, lettuce, dry beans, and peas.

Manganese deficiency states are rare in humans. Increases in prothrombin time and a bleeding diathesis unresponsive to vitamin K have been reported in manganese deficiency. Lack of manganese in animals has been found to cause improper formation of bone and cartilage, gonadal dysfunction, a decrease in the body's ability to use sugar properly, and growth problems.

Because manganese deficiency is rare, a RDA has not been established. However, a daily intake of 2 to 5 milligrams (mg) is considered to be satisfactory for most individuals.

Manganese toxicity may be manifested by an encephalitis like syndrome, psychosis and pneumoconiosis. Miners who inhale large quantities of manganese develop asthenia, loss of appetite, apathy, headache, impotence, leg cramps, and speech disturbances on chronic exposure to manganese.

Additional manganese information and selected food sources are available at:
http://www.nlm.nih.gov/medlineplus (search "manganese")
http://www.foodstandards.gov.uk

6.6.8 Molybdenum

Molybdenum is an essential trace antioxidant mineral that serves as a part of enzyme systems that are required for normal growth and health.

Peas, beans, cereal products, leafy vegetables, and milk are good food sources for molybdenum. The amount of molybdenum in foods depends on the soil in which the food is grown.

A deficiency of molybdenum is rare. However, if the body does not obtain enough molybdenum, certain enzymes are affected, and this may lead to a build up of unwanted substances and a deficiency state.

The IOM has not established a RDA for molybdenum. Daily intakes of 75 to 250 micrograms, however, are considered sufficient for most adults. Missing molybdenum intake for one or more days is no cause for concern since it takes some time for the body to become seriously low in this trace mineral.

Molybdenum may worsen copper deficiency. In cases of kidney or liver disease, higher blood levels of molybdenum may increase the chance of adverse effects.

Side effects of excessive molybdenum intake may include joint pain, side or lower back or stomach pain, and/or swelling of the feet or lower legs. Such side effects are rarely seen in individuals consuming a high dietary content of molybdenum.

Additional molybdenum information and selected food sources are available at:
http://www.acu-cell.com/vmo.html
http://www.foodstandards.gov.uk

6.6.9 Selenium

Selenium is an essential trace mineral that plays a key role in concert with antioxidants to protect cells against the effects of free radicals produced during cellular metabolism. This is part of the system that the body uses to control levels of free radicals and cell damage that can contribute to the development of chronic diseases. Selenium also is essential for normal functioning of the immune system and thyroid gland.

Plant foods are the major dietary sources of selenium. Selenium in the soil determines in a great measure, the amount of selenium in the plant foods grown in that area. It can also be found in some meats and seafood. Nuts, especially Brazil nuts and walnuts, also are good sources of selenium.

Selenium deficiency is most commonly seen in parts of Russia and China where the selenium content in the soil is low and selenium intake is inadequate. Deficiency is linked to a disorder called Keshan Disease characterized by an enlarged heart and poor heart function. Thyroid function also may be altered in deficiency states because selenium is essential for the synthesis of thyroid hormone. Selenium deficiency also may worsen the effects of any iodine deficiency on thyroid function. Adequate selenium intake helps protect against neurological effects of iodine deficiency.

Patients requiring total parenteral nutrition (TPN) as their sole source of nutrition may develop selenium deficiency unless they are supplemented with selenium. Several gastrointestinal disorders characterized by malabsorption also may decrease the absorption resulting in selenium deficiency. These include

• severe gastrointestinal disorders that may impair absorption

• removal of over 50% of the intestines or gastric bypass surgery.

Mortality from colorectal, lung, and prostate cancers is reported to be lower in individuals with higher selenium blood levels or intakes. Also in areas of the United States with low soil selenium levels, the incidence of skin cancer (non-melanoma) is reported to be significantly higher.

Selenium supplementation (200 micrograms daily) is reported to reduce total mortality, as well as mortality from colorectal, lung and prostate cancers but not the recurrence of skin cancer. However, not all studies have shown a relationship between selenium and cancer and more studies are needed for clarification.

Available evidence also indicates a potential basis for the use of selenium as an antioxidant in the prevention of cardiovascular disease. However, there is insufficient evidence available to recommend selenium supplements for the prevention of cardiovascular disease at this time.

Patients with rheumatoid arthritis are reported to have reduced selenium levels in their blood as well as low selenium intake in their diet. Selenium, as an antioxidant, may help control the levels of free radicals produced in the inflammatory process in rheumatoid arthritis, and help relieve symptoms and favorably alter the course of the disease. However, further research is needed before selenium supplements can be recommended for individuals with rheumatoid arthritis.

Mice given a diet deficient in selenium and exposed to a human influenza virus develop a more severe case of the flu and lung damage compared to those fed adequate amounts of this trace element, suggesting that selenium deficiency can increase the virulence of viruses. Also, normally harmless coxsackie virus apparently mutates into a heart damaging pathogen in selenium deficient mice. This research suggests that selenium may offer certain protection against harmful effects of virus infections but this needs to be confirmed in human subjects.

Selenium toxicity is uncommon in the United State. However, high intake can result in a condition called selenosis, characterized by gastrointestinal upsets, hair loss, nerve damage, and white blotchy nails. The IOM has set a safe, tolerable upper level (UL) for selenium at 400 micrograms per day for adults.

Additional selenium information and selected food sources are available at:
http://lpi.oregonstate.edu/infocenter/minerals/selenium/index.html
http://www.nlm.nih.gov/medlineplus (search "selenium")
http://www.foodstandards.gov.uk

6.6.10 Zinc

Zinc is an essential trace mineral antioxidant that plays a role in activity of around 100 enzymes involved in the body. It is found in almost every cell/tissue/organ and not only supports a healthy immune system and wound healing, it maintains the sense of smell and taste. It is needed for DNA syntheses, and supports normal growth and development. Zinc is found in a wide variety of foods such as oysters, red meat and poultry, beans, nuts, certain seafood, whole grains, dairy products, and fortified breakfast cereals. Absorption of zinc is greater from a diet high in animal, compared to plant, proteins. Phytates in plant foods such as whole grain breads, cereals, legumes, etc. can decrease zinc absorption.

Deficiency can occur when zinc intake is insufficient to meet daily needs, the mineral is poorly absorbed, there are increased losses, or the body's requirement increases. Signs of zinc deficiency may include loss of appetite, diarrhea, eye lesions, growth retardation, hair loss, impotence, and skin lesions. Weight loss, delayed wound healing, mental lethargy, taste abnormalities also may occur.

Supplementation of zinc in the diet may be required in certain circumstances, namely.

• vegetarians require significantly more zinc because of the lower absorption from plant food.

• 30% to 50% of alcoholics may have a deficiency because alcohol decreases the absorption of zinc and increases loss in the urine. Also, alcoholics may not eat an acceptable variety or amount of food, and their intake of zinc may be inadequate

• loss of zinc due to chronic diarrhea

• digestive disorders such as sprue, Crohn's disease, and other intestinal disorders that may cause malabsorption of zinc

Moderate to severe zinc deficiency can depress immune function. Development and activation of T-lymphocytes, white blood cells that help fight infection, require zinc for activation. Zinc supplements in patients with depressed immune function increase the numbers of circulating T-lymphocytes and their ability to fight infection. Zinc supplements in deficient individuals also may shorten the course of infectious diarrhea, and may help heal skin ulcers and bed sores in patients.

Recent research indicates that a supplement mixture of zinc and antioxidant vitamins, may prevent further vision loss in people with age related macular degeneration

Additional zinc information and selected food sources are available at:
http://www.cc.nih.gov/ccc/supplements/zinc.html
http://lpi.oregonstate.edu/info/minerals/zinc/index.html.
http://www.nlm.nih.gov/medlineplus (search "zinc")
http://www.foodstandards.gov.uk

6.7 Unclassified Trace Minerals

Boron is the only unclassified trace mineral discussed in this section. Insufficient information is available on other trace minerals such as nickel, silicon and vanadium and they will not be considered further in this book.

6.7.1 Boron

Boron is an essential micronutrient for higher plant life. However, insufficient evidence exists to officially designate boron as essential for human health at this time.

Available research suggests that boron may be useful in trace amounts in humans for the formation and maintenance of healthy bones and teeth. Results of studies indicate that boron may play a key role in bone metabolism (e.g. calcification) and thus could be useful in the prevention of osteoporosis and tooth decay. Boron is reported to enhance the absorption of calcium, magnesium, and play a role in the metabolism of calcium, magnesium and phosphorous. In addition, it appears to raise plasma estrogen and testosterone levels, and aid estrogen in its role in helping convert vitamin D into its active form, calcitriol. Postmenopausal women are reported to lose 40% less calcium and one third less magnesium plus somewhat less phosphorous in their urine after 8 days of supplementing their diet with 3 mg/day of boron. Storage of boron in the parathyroid glands suggests further possible interaction with parathyroid hormone, calcium, and bone.

Recent studies have shown that the risk of prostate cancer falls as the intake of boron climbs. Prostate cancer risk for men consuming 1.8 mg/day of boron has been found to be less than one third of those with an intake of 0.9 mg/day. Almonds, coffee, certain fruits, nuts, and red wine, rich in boron may reduce the risk of prostate cancer in men. A recent study showed that men who consumed the greatest amount of boron were 64% less likely to develop prostate cancer.

Boron deficient rats are reported to be susceptible to certain autoimmune disorders. And boron has been found to be protective against such disorders presumably by blocking of the activation of T-suppressor and T-helper cells considered to be important in the autoimmune chain reactions. This effect is reported to occur at doses estimated to be equivalent to 2 mg/day of boron in a person's diet. This evidence suggests a possible role for boron in human autoimmune disorders such as rheumatoid arthritis, etc.

Although boron is abundantly common in various food sources, American adults are reported to consume, on average, only around 1 mg/day of boron in their diet (while a number of other nations have a much higher intake). A glass of wine, a small handful of peanuts, or a serving of noncitrus fruit each offers close to 0.5 mg of boron. Avocado (5 oz.) is reported to provide 3.0 mg, kidney beans (5 oz) 2.0 mg, peanuts (2 oz) 1.0 mg, almonds (2 oz) 1.0 mg, and prunes (2 oz) 1.0 mg. Plants, green leafy vegetables, legumes, grapes, raisins and apples also are considered to be reasonably good food sources for boron. Intake from food sources of between 2-3 mg/day of boron is reported to be reasonable safe and well tolerated. The upper intake (UL) limit may be around 20 mg/day.

Excess boron intake may result in adverse reactions and/or toxicity. This may be manifested by gastrointestinal disturbances, anemia, skin and hair loss, metabolic imbalance (acidosis) convulsions, and cardiac arrest.

Boron can be very toxic and lethal at high doses. The fact that boric acid, sprinkled around the house in powdered form, is lethal to cockroaches attests to its toxicity.

Additional boron information and selected food sources are available at:
http://www.webmd.com (search "boron" for information)
http://www.foodstandards.gov.uk

6.8 Multiple Vitamin/Mineral Supplement

Major medical organizations/experts appear to agree that the best way to obtain recommended amounts of all essential vitamins and minerals is through a nutritionally balanced diet. However, many individuals do not know what constitutes a nutritionally balanced diet or follow one consistently, and therefor may be deficient in one or more ways, and benefit from taking a daily multiple vitamin/mineral supplement. Thus, an essential multiple vitamin/mineral supplement may be indicated especially in those adults who:

- don't eat the recommended 5 to 9 servings a day of fruits and vegetables

- are 55 and older, when health problems may contribute to an inadequate dietary intake and poor absorption

- are on vegetarian, low caloric, or special diets that limits intake

- have a disease of the gallbladder, intestine, or pancreas or surgery of the gastrointestinal tract, etc. that may limit the ability to digest and/or absorb sufficient amounts of essential vitamins/minerals

- drink more than 1-2 drinks/day of alcoholic beverages that may impair absorption/utilization or increase excretion of vitamins and/or minerals

- are not able to obtain recommended amounts from food for any other reason

Choosing a vitamin/mineral supplement, should not be considered a substitute for replacement for nutrients found in whole foods and needed for a nutritionally balanced diet. However, once the decision is made, the vitamin/mineral supplement should:

- be one that provides 100% of the Daily Value (DV) of essential vitamins/minerals instead of one that provides "megadoses" or significantly less than the DV

- have USP on the label indicating that it meets standards for disintegration, dissolution, purity, and strength established by the U.S. Pharmacopeia.

- not be one marketed as "natural" since such are generally regarded as no different from the synthetic varieties and may cost more

- not contain added herbs, enzymes, or amino acids which may only add cost but not provide significant extra benefit

- have an appropriate expiration date on the label (as supplements can lose potency over time, especially in hot and humid climates).

- be one that is appropriate for medical condition/nutritional status of the consumer

- have compatibility with any prescription drugs, herbs, or other medications being taken

Too many/too much of vitamin/mineral supplements can be detrimental to health, especially if taken for long periods of time without medical supervision. For example, recent evidence indicates that high intake of supplemental chromium picolinate may cause genetic damage whereas other forms of chromium in doses of 10 milligrams per day or less are considered safe in this regard. More than 1,000 milligrams per day of vitamin C, 1,500 milligrams/day of calcium, or 17 milligrams/day of iron may cause adverse effects in some individuals. Beta carotene may produce irreversible harmful effects in smokers when taken long term and in high doses. Manganese, nicotinic acid (niacin), zinc, and phosphorous also can be harmful in high doses over the long term. Numerous other examples also suggest "consumer beware".

Information regarding the safety of 34 vitamins and minerals is available at:

- Food Standards Agency

  http://www.foodstandards.gov.uk

- American Society for Nutritional Sciences

  http://www.nutrition.org

- US Food and Drug Administration

  http://www.fda.gov

7. Author's List/Key Web Sources

The Author's selection of 30 key Web Resources used in this book are arranged alphabetically with content outlined in sections 7.1-7.30 respectively. Each of the Web Resources also provides a Search site to obtain additional information on nutrition and health topics of interest.

7.1 AlltheWeb
http://www.alltheweb.com

AlltheWeb is a European international search engine operated by Fast Search and Transfer (FAST), the leading provider of the real time search and filter technology solutions that are behind the scenes at some of the world's best known companies with the most demanding search problems.

AlltheWeb combines one of the largest with one of the most powerful search features that allows one to find "almost anything". It:

* indexes over 2.1 billion Web pages, as well as tens of millions of PDF and MS Word files.

* scans the "entire Web" every 7-11 days to ensure content is fresh and there are no broken links

* supports searching in 49 different languages

* provides News search, and up to the minute news from thousands of news sources all across the globe indexing hundreds of stories every minute.

In addition, it is reported to have one of the most sophisticated advanced search features and can provide one with a large number of key nutrition and health links/reports.

7.2 American Dietetic Association
http://www.eatright.org
http://www.eatright.org/Public

The ADA, with around 70,000 members, is the nation's largest organization of food and nutrition professionals. ADA serves the public by promoting optimal nutrition, health and well being.

"Healthy Eating, Healthy You" is the theme for this year's (2003) National Nutrition Month. Being healthy begins with knowing what foods your body needs for fuel, growth and health.

ADA provides click on sites for information on:

- About ADA
- ADA Journal
- ADA Position Papers/Position Categories including ones on
  - Aging
  - Diets/dieting
  - Food technology/food safety
  - Healthcare/reform
  - Medical education
  - Public health
- Find a Nutrition Professional
- Research Summaries for the Public

7.3 American Heart Association
http://www.americanheart.org
http://www.americanheart.org/
presenter.jhml?=1200000

The AHA is a large lay and professional organization devoted to nutrition and health, cardiovascular disease and stroke. Their national center is located in Dallas, Texas with 15 affiliate offices throughout the US. Combined efforts involve the work of millions of volunteers and supporters dedicated to the primary task of reducing disability and death from cardiovascular diseases and stroke. It provides current, reliable information to the public and professionals on nutrition and health.

7.4 American Medical Association
http://www.ama-assn.org

The AMA is one of the nation's leaders in promoting professionalism in medicine. Its mission is to promote sound nutrition and health, and medicine for the betterment of public health. The Consumer Health Information site allows one to learn how to improve nutrition and health with easy-to-understand, current, reliable information.

7.5 Food and Drug Administration
http://www.fda.gov
http://cfsan.fda.gov

The FDA regulates food, nutrition and dietary supplements. Food and nutrition matters are evaluated/regulated by the FDA Center for Food Safety and Applied Nutrition (CFSAN). Direct access to their nutrition site is available at:
http://cfsan.fda.gov

7.6 Food Standards Agency
http://www.foodstandards.gov.uk

The Food Standards Agency is an independent food safety watchdog set up by an Act of Parliament in the United Kingdom in 2000 to protect the public's health and consumer interests in relation to food. The FSA represents the UK government on food safety and standards issues in the European Union.

FSA Food Directory A-Z, a click on link, is packed with food safety and healthy eating advice on a great number of topics of interest. For information on vitamins and minerals, click first on "Diet and Health", and then on "Vitamins and Minerals". The information given is aimed at adults. The direct Web site access for this information is:
http://www.food.gov/uk/healthiereating/vitaminsminerals/vitaminsaz

The "Diet and Health" click on link also provides information on food intolerance, diet and weight, food myths debunked, food related conditions, ask an expert, and other key topics of interest.

7.7 Google.com
http://www.google.com

GOOGLE is one of the largest, fastest search engines, capable of searching "the entire world wide Web". A number of different language tools are made available for searches/translations in various languages offered. Google currently searches over 3 billion web pages worldwide. A large number of current, reliable nutrition and health links/reports are provided.

7.8 Harvard School of Public Health
http://www.hsph.harvard.edu/nutritionsource

This nutrition and health site is maintained by the Department of Nutrition at the Harvard School of Public Health. The mission of the Department of Nutrition is to improve human health through enhanced nutrition. The department strives to accomplish this goal through research aimed at improved understanding of how diet influences health, the dissemination of new knowledge about nutrition to health professionals and the public, the development of nutritional strategies, and the education of researchers and practitioners.

Click on information sites are provided for:

- Interpreting News on Diet
- Carbohydrates
- Fats and Cholesterol
- Protein
- Fiber
- Fruits and Vegetables
- Calcium and Milk
- Vitamins
- Healthy Weight
- Food Pyramids
- More Information

7.9 Health.gov
http://www.health.gov
http://www.health.gov/dietary guidelines

Health.gov is a portal to the Web sites of a number of health initiatives and activities of the US Department of Health and Human Services and other Federal departments and agencies. Features a click on site for a new report on "Steps to a Healthier US".

"Nutrition and Your Health: Dietary Guidelines for Americans", a joint effort of the Office of Disease Prevention, Department of Health and Human Service (IIIIS), and the Center for Nutrition Policy and Promotion (CNPP), US Department of Agriculture (USDA) dated May 2000 also is available online at:
http://www.health.gov/dietaryguidelines.

Principles of the Dietary Guidelines discussed include links/information on:

- aim for fitness
- aim for a healthy weight

- be physically active each day

- build a healthy nutritional base

- let the Pyramid guide your food choices

- choose a variety of grains daily, especially whole grains

- choose a variety of fruits, vegetables, seeds and nuts daily

- keep food safe to eat

- select foods sensibly

- adopt a diet low in saturated fats, trans fats, and cholesterol, and moderate in total fat

- moderate intake of sugars/refined carbohydrates in the diet

- prepare food with less salt

- drink alcoholic beverages in moderation or not at all

Selected additional US Government Resources, links/information also are provided.

7.10 Health on the Net Foundation
http://www.hon.ch

HON is regarded as one of the most respected nonprofit Web sites for medical/nutrition information on the Web. It is a Swiss foundation operating out of Geneva, Switzerland with generous support of the local Geneva government, the University Hospitals of Geneva, and the Swiss Institute of Bioinformatics. HON's distinguished guiding council members and Web team hail from several European countries and the USA. Information is provided in English, French, German, Spanish or Portuguese.

Distinguishing features of this Web sit include:

- two widely used medical search tools, MedHunt and HonSelect

- HON code of Conduct for selection of authoritative, trustworthy, Web based nutrition/health information

In addition, HON offers free access to Medline and PubMed at the National Library of Medicine, and the ability to search these large compendiums of articles on nutrition and health.

7.11 Institute of Medicine
http://www.iom.edu

For science based advice about issues of medicine and public health, the nation's leaders turn to an institution that was created specifically for this purpose, the Institute of Medicine. The IOM, a nonprofit organization chartered in 1970 as a component of the National Academy of Sciences, provides a public service outside the framework of government to insure independent guidance on matters of nutrition, health, and medicine. The IOM's mission is to advance and disseminate scientific knowledge and improve medicine, nutrition and human health. It provides objective, timely, authoritative information and advice concerning health and science policy to government, the corporate sector, the health professions, and the public. The IOM is organized into 9 oversight boards, one of which is the Food and Nutrition Board (FNB) that provides current, comprehensive, authoritative key reports on food, nutrition and health.

The FNB direct access Web site can be found at:
http://www.iom.edu/IOM/IOM/IOMHOME.
nsf/pages/Food+and+Nutrition+Board
http://www.iom.edu/board.asp?ID=3788

7.12 Iowa State University/Extension
http://www.extension.iastate.edu/nutrition

Food systems are changing and consumers may now choose among organically and traditionally grown foods. The purposes of the Iowa State University Extension (ISUE) are to help consumers understand new food choices and evaluate them in relation to individual values and health goals.

Key publications available from ISUE include:

- *The Health Value of Fruits and Vegetables*

- *What You Need to Know About Health Benefits of Functional Foods*

- *What You Need to Know About Health Claims on Foods*

- *What You Need to Know About New Food Words-Phytochemicals, Functional Foods, and Nutraceuticals*

A key phytochemicals report provided is:

- *Phytochemicals—Vitamins of the Future*

    Ohio State University Extension Fact Sheet
    http://ohioline.ag.ohio-state.edu/hyg-fact/5000/5050.html

7.13 Mayo Clinic
http://www.mayo.edu

The Mayo Clinic is an exemplary nonprofit organization located in Rochester, Minnesota with branches in Arizona and Florida. More than 2,000 physicians and 35,000 allied health staff, scientists, researchers and other professionals work in the Mayo system. Current comprehensive and reliable nutrition and health information is made available through their database and key links to other sources. Information is available in both English and Spanish languages.

7.14 Medline
http://medline.cos.com

Medline, compiled by the National Library of Medicine, is the world's most comprehensive library resource containing around 11 million records from over 7000 different publications from 1965 to today. Information made available is updated weekly. Medline provides both abstracts and full article publications.

Medline also may be accessed via the National Library of Medicine and Health on the Net at:

http://www.nlm.nih.gov
http://www.hon.ch.

Health on the Net Foundation (HON) provides free access to Medline.

7.15 Medlineplus
http://www.nlm.nih.gov/medlineplus

Medlineplus is a service of the National Library of Medicine (the world's largest medical library) and the National Institutes of Health (a trusted source of medical information) utilizing their online databases involving over 11 million documents. Medlineplus does not accept any advertising on their Web site nor do they endorse any company or product. Medlineplus provides summaries and references on nutrition and health topics of interest plus links to further information.

Also, Medline may be searched for recent research reports by clicking on the "Vitamin and Mineral Supplements" link for information on this topic. The direct access website is:

http://www.nlm.nih.gov/medlineplus/vitaminsandmineralsupplements.html

For information on nutrition and health go to their "Health Information" link and click on any topic A-Z of interest.

In addition you may click on links provided for dictionaries, encyclopedias, and glossaries that provide spellings and definitions of words/terms.

7.16 National Cancer Institute
http://www.cancer.gov

The National Cancer Institute (NCI) of the National Institute of Health (NIH) is the premier US government effort and resource regarding cancer. It provides current, comprehensive, reliable, and useful information for patients and health care professionals on nutrition and cancer.

7.17 National Center for Chronic Disease Prevention and Health Promotion
http://www.cdc.gov/nccdphp/dnpa
http://www.cdc.gov

The Centers for Disease Control (CDC) serves as the national focus for developing and applying disease prevention and control, environmental health, and promotional and educational activities designed to improve the health of people in the United States and abroad.

One of the major CDC centers is the National Center for Chronic Disease Prevention and Health Promotion (NCCDPHP). The Division of Nutrition and Physical Activity (DNPA) at NCCDPHP addresses the role of nutrition and physical activity in health and the prevention and control of chronic diseases. DNPA is organized into the: 1) Chronic Disease Nutrition Branch, 2) Maternal Nutrition Branch, and 3) Physical Activity and Health Branch.

Click on the "Nutrition" site for relevant information provided.

7.18 National Institute on Aging
http://www.nia.nih.gov

NIA leads a broad scientific effort to understand the nature of aging and to extend the healthy, active years of life. It is the primary federal agency on Alzheimer's disease research.

One of NIA's key missions is to improve nutrition, health, and well being of older Americans through research, and specifically to:

- support and conduct high quality research on the:
  - aging process
  - age related diseases
  - special problems and needs of the aged

- develop and maintain state-of-the art resources to accelerate aging research progress

7.19 National Institutes of Health
http://www.nih.gov

The NIH comprises 27 Institutes and Centers, and is one of the leading federal research efforts concerning nutrition and health research in the United States.

A key "Consensus Statement 60: Diet and Exercise in Non-Insulin Dependent Diabetes Mellitus" is available at:
http://www.consenus.nih.gov/cons/060/060_statement.htm

7.20 National Institute of Health/Clinical Center
http://www.cc.nih.gov
http://www.cc.nih.gov/ccc/suppplements/intro.html

The National Institute of Health/Clinical Center is on the forefront of medical discovery and provides current, comprehensive, reliable and useful information on nutrition and health. It provides fact sheets entitled "Facts About Dietary Supplements" on such topics as vitamin A, B-6, B-12, D, E and folate, iron, magnesium, selenium, and zinc. These fact sheets are developed in conjunction with the NIH Office of Dietary Supplements and are consistent with the Dietary Guidelines for Americans. The direct access website for this supplement information is: http://www.cc.nih.gov/ccc/supplements/intro.html

7.21 National Library of Medicine
http://www.nlm.nih.gov

NLM is the world's largest medical library with click on links to Medline, Medlineplus, and PubMed. Key links to nutrition and health information also are provided.

The PubMed site provides abstracts of articles and references. Medlineplus provides reports and references. Medline provides full text of articles plus references on topics of interest.

7.22 Nutrition.Gov
http://www.nutrition.gov/home/index.php3

Nutrition.Gov is a premier US Government resource for current, comprehensive, reliable and useful nutrition information. Click on links are provided for nutrition and health information on:

- Consumption
- Dietary Guidelines
- Dietary Supplements
- Education Programs
- Food Pyramid

- Food Labels
- Healthy Eating
- Nutrients

Additional click on information sites are available for "Food Safety", and "Lifecycle Issues".

7.23 Nutrition.Org/American Society for Nutritional Sciences
http://www.nutrition.org

The American Society for Nutritional Sciences publishes the Journal of Nutrition, and services their Web site, Nutrition.Org. A site is provided for "Search for Articles" in the Journal of Nutrition 1997-present.

Click on "Nutrient Information" and the "Food Guide Pyramid" for information on:

* Food nutrients A-Z

* Vitamins and Minerals

* Phytochemicals (Phytonutrients)

* Electrolytes (Sodium, Chloride, Potassium)

* Carbohydrates, Fats, and Protein

Direct access to food nutrient information is available at:
http://www.nutrition.org/nutinfo

7.24 Office of Dietary Supplements
http://dietary-supplements.info.nih.gov

ODS, a branch of the National Institute of Health, supports research and disseminates information regarding dietary supplements. Click on links are provided for:

* What Are Dietary Supplements

* Dietary Reference Intakes (DRIs)

* Recommended Dietary Allowances (RDAs)

* fact sheets

- publications

- links for consumers

- links for scientists

DRIs are available for:

- macronutrients

- minerals

- vitamins

Reports are provided on:

- calcium and related nutrients

- dietary antioxidants and related compounds

- folate and other B vitamins

- macronutrients (carbohydrates, fat and protein)

- vitamins A and K and selected micronutrients

"Health Information" and "Research" click on sites are also available.

7.25 Tufts Nutritional Navigator
http://navigator.tufts.edu

TNN is a rating guide for nutrition and health Web sites. It was developed by the Tufts University Gerald and Dorothy Friedman School of Nutritional Science and Policy, a respected academic center for nutritional information excellence, and is underwritten by a grant from Kraft Foods.

TNN's rating and review guide allows one to: 1) quickly find nutritional information on the Web which is best suited to the needs of the inquirer, 2) sort through volumes of nutritional reports to find those most useful, and 3) have confidence and trust in the information obtained. Web sites featured are reviewed by Tuft's nutrition experts who apply rating and evaluation criteria developed by Tuft's University Nutrition Navigator Advisory Board, a prestigious panel of leading US and Canadian nutrition experts.

Information on this Web site is updated quarterly to ensure ratings take into consideration new information. Key links/information sites are featured for timely information.

7.26 USDA Center for Nutrition Policy Promotion
http://www.usda.gov/cnpp

The Center for Nutrition Policy Promotion (CNPP) was created by the US Department of Agriculture (USDA) to be the focal point where scientific research provides key nutrition and health information to the American Public and others. CNPP carries out its mission by:

• developing and coordinating nutrition policy within the USDA

• investigating techniques for effective nutrition communication

• evaluating the nutrient content of the US food supply

• preparing periodic updates on the cost of family food plans

• assessing cost effectiveness of government sponsored nutrition programs concerning food consumption, expenditures, behavior and nutritional status.

Click on links/reports featured include:

• ABCs of Dietary Guidelines

• USDA Supports 5 to 9 a Day for Better Health

• How Much Are You Eating

• Dietary Guidelines for Americans 2000

- Interactive Healthy Index

- Recipes and Tips for Healthy, Thrifty Meals

- Nutritional Insights

- Food Guide Pyramid

- Nutrition and Aging

- Dietary Behavior: Why We Choose the Foods We Eat

Links to other Web Resources, reports and information on nutrition and health are provided.

7.27 USDA Food and Nutrition Information Center
http://www.nal.usda.gov/fnic

The USDA Food and Nutrition Information Center (FNIC) is located at the National Agricultural Library (NAL), a part of the US Department of Agriculture (USDA) and the Agricultural Research Service (ARS). FNIC has a Cooperative Agreement with the University of Maryland's Department of Nutrition and Food Science in the College of Agriculture and Natural Resources. FNIC's mission is to collect and disseminate current, comprehensive, reliable and useful information about food and human nutrition. It is a leader in online global nutrition and health information provided by registered dieticians/scientists on food, human nutrition and health.

Click on topics:

- Topic A-Z
- FNIC resources links
- Dietary supplements

- Food Guide Pyramid
- FNIC databases
- Consumer Corner

- Food composition
- Dietary Guidelines

- Vitamins/Minerals

Key information is provided on vitamins and minerals. A click on site is provided for Dietary Reference Intakes (DRIs), Recommended Dietary Allowance (RDAs) and Dietary Supplements (DSs). The direct access Web site for this information is: http://www.nal.usda.gov/fnic/etext/000068.html

7.28 USDA Nutrient Data Laboratory/ Agricultural Research Service
http://www.nal.usda.gov/fnic/foodcomp
http://www.nal.usda.gov/fnic/foodcomp/Data/
SR15/sr15.html

The NDL/ARS is part of the USDA and functions as part of a Cooperative Agreement with the University of Maryland's Department of Nutrition and Food Science in the College of Agriculture and Natural Resources.

It provides information sites for:

- About Nutrient Data Laboratory

- Food Composition

- USDA National Nutrient Database for Standard Reference reports on:

  - single nutrients
  - nutritive value of foods
  - flavonoids
  - isoflavones
  - carotenoids

  - vitamin K
  - trans fatty acids
  - sugar
  - key foods

The NDL is responsible for developing authoritative nutrient databases that contain food composition values for the nation's food supply. However, with almost 6000 food items in the database, analyzing every food item for every nutrient and meeting user requirements is impossible. Consequently, priorities have been established, and nutrient values for key food (those that contribute up to 75% of any one nutrient) are being used to set priorities for nutrient analyses under the National Food and Nutrient Analyses Program. (see http://www.nal.usda.gov/fnic/foodcomp/Bulletins/keyfoods.htm).

Click on sites are made available for:

- Information
  - How to Get Information from NDL
  - FAQs (Frequently Asked Questions)
  - Food composition and nutrition
  - Articles by NDL staff
  - Glossary
  - Measurement conversion tables
  - Compiling food composition data for 110 years

- What's New
  - database for the flavonoid content of selected foods
  - classic USDA food composition publications
  - oxalic acid content of selected vegetables
  - key foods (providing up to 75% of any one nutrient)
  - selenium content of foods
  - vitamin D content of food.

7.29 USDA Phytonutrient Laboratory
http://www.barc.usda.gov/bhnrc/pl

The mission of the USDA Phytonutrient Laboratory is to:

- characterize phytonutrients present in foods and delineate their metabolism in humans

- clarify the role(s) of these chemical compounds in animal and human health

- provide information relative to the intake of fruits, vegetables, and grains, and their phytonutrient content.

Click on links are provided for: 1) human nutrition research, 2) databases, 3) frequently asked questions and answers and related links.

The USDA Fruit Laboratory site can be found at:
http://www.barc.usda.gov/psi/fl/fl.html

Frequently Asked Questions and Answers on phytonutrients can be found at:
http://www.barc.usda.gov/bhnrc/pl/pl_faq.html

Common questions and answers covered include:

- What are phytonutrients and where are they found

- What are the major classes of phytonutrients

- How do phytonutrients protect against disease

- What is the evidence that fruit and vegetable consumption protects human health

- Are Americans eating enough fruits and vegetables

- What is the present state of phytonutrient research

7.30 WebMD
http://www.webmd.com

WebMD is a for profit corporation providing services that help consumers, healthcare workers, and physicians navigate the complexity of the health system and the Web, making current, comprehensive and reliable nutrition and health information available to users.

8. Searching the Web

Many books have been written on how to use/search the Web. One may be obtained from a local public library or bookstore. Or one recently published by the author entitled: "Web Health Information Resource Guide: For Consumers, Healthcare Providers, Patients and Physicians" published in 2001 by Author's Choice Press, iuniverse.com, may be used. The Web page for the book is:
http://www.webspawner.com/users/webhealthdoc. It can be "browsed" on the publisher's website at: http://www.iuniverse.com.

A number of commercial services such as AOL, MSN, Netscape, Road Runner and Yahoo, as well as others, provide easy, reliable, and relatively inexpensive access to the Internet/Web via a computer. If one does not have a computer, a local public, college or university library can provide one to connect to the Internet/Web at no cost and little effort. If needed the local reference librarian can provide instruction on how to use the Web to facilitate a search. Should a computer not be available, a Web TV or similar device can be hooked up to a TV set at home, or a hand held device may be used to connect to the Internet/Web. Once connected, the Author's List/Key Web Resources provided in Chapter 7 may be used for a search. These Web resources are arranged alphabetically, along with a brief outline of the kinds of information available on each, for ease of reference and selection.

Not all information made available on the Web should be considered current, comprehensive, reliable or useful. Be selective and use due diligence in any search, and use of information obtained. A good way to select appropriate Web resources is to use guidelines in choosing them. Such guidelines may be obtained from a number of sources such as:

American Medical Association
http://www.ama-assn.org/ama/pub/category/1905.html

Health on the Net Foundation
http://www.hon.ch (go to "HON Code of Conduct")

Criteria used by different organizations in selecting reliable Web resources
varies. Nevertheless, using the guidelines developed by the two previously
mentioned organizations, or others, should provide reliable Web resource
information.

The Author's List/Key Web Resources summarized in Chapter 7 is a person-
ally reviewed selection providing "current, comprehensive, reliable and useful"
information on nutrition and health for the vast majority of consumers,
healthcare providers, patients and physicians. In addition, other key Web sites
are included in the text of this book, referencing key points of information.

The World Wide Web currently is estimated at well over 3 billion pages, and
still growing rapidly. When searching the Web with a search engine such as
Google or AlltheWeb, one is not searching it directly as this is not feasible at
this time. The Web is the totality of all the Web pages and documents that
reside on computers, called servers, worldwide, and a computer cannot locate
and search them directly. All one can do with a computer is to go to one of a
number of intermediate resources that contain selected and organized Web
pages and databases. Thus, via AlltheWeb or Google, for example, one merely
searches their intermediate resources/databases and they provide the links to
the Web pages needed to complete a search. One then can click on these
links/Web pages and retrieve information pertaining to a particular search.

Google or AlltheWeb can provide one with a reasonably "complete" search on
nutrition and health topics of interest, usually in less than a second or so.
However, then one is left with the very difficult task of reviewing all the links/
Web pages/reports/information found in order to find the ones that are current, comprehensive, reliable, and useful. This is not only difficult and time
consuming but also usually well beyond the capability of most readers to
accomplish in a reasonable period of time.

To simplify matters, the author has carefully selected and assembled the
Author's List/Key Web Resources and provided them in alphabetical order for

ease of reference. The main nutrition and health content of each of the Web Resources is outlined briefly to facilitate selection of those most likely to provide the information being sought. Each Web Resource provides a Search site that may be used to obtain additional nutrition and health information on topics of interest from their database.

Remember that the Web is growing rapidly and is in a constant state of flux, updating, and reorganization. Web Resources may change their names and/or Web site addresses, formats, content and categorization of information offered. If for any reason the Web address chosen from the Author's List, or the book's text, doesn't work, search the Web Resource itself and use their Search site for the desired information. If there still are problems connecting, use another Search Engine to access the Web site, Web Resource or nutrition topic in question.

Keep in mind that various Web Resources use different methods to search the Web to compile their databases and information offered. Also, each Web Resource organizes and categorizes information differently, some better and easier to use than others. Thus, searches using different Web Resources or topics may provide results that differ and need to be reconciled by further work. And Web pages/reports may be removed or not be available for a number of reasons. So search accordingly.

For the most part, the information found via the Author's List may be regarded as reasonably current, comprehensive, reliable and useful in most respects, but not necessarily all. Thus, information obtained from any one source on the Web should not necessarily be relied upon. Unlike medical/scientific articles published in peer reviewed professional journals, there is no guarantee that the information obtained from any Web Resource will be useful. Also, keep in mind that Web Resources are not uniformly reliable in all aspects of all information offered at all times. Therefore, Web Resources chosen should be appropriate, and information obtained from at least 2-3 or more should be compared, before reaching any conclusions/decisions in consultation with a healthcare provider/physician. Even in the amazing world of the Web, a second or third opinion, is still considered to be worthwhile.

One also needs to consider that even in the case of scientific, evidence based information from well controlled clinical trials, there are problems in terms of what the data collected/results mean. Clinical study evidence necessarily is subject to interpretation and application and, as such, is a subjective process. Everyone is biased to some degree in one way or another not only in obtaining, but also in interpreting and applying information, evidence based or not. Words, phrases, statistics, conclusions, etc. mean different things to different people at different times and places, depending on "where one is coming from". For example, even in the case of a long standing document such as the Constitution of the United States written by "great minds", people, lawyers, judges, and even the Supreme Court continue to debate, argue about, and have great difficulty interpreting and applying, the so-called "original intent" of our founding fathers and authors of this great document.

Nevertheless, available evidence indicates that there are significant improvements in our understanding of nutrition that can significantly improve health and longevity. Therefore, take charge, control and responsibility for becoming informed about nutrition, and live a healthier, happier, longer and more productive/enjoyable life.

About the Author

Eugene A. De Felice, M.D., is a recognized author, educator, and Distinguished Clinical Professor of Medicine who is listed in the prestigious Marquis': 1) Who's Who in Medicine and Healthcare, 2) Who's Who in America, and 3) Who's Who in the World. He is the author of numerous medical/scientific articles published in professional journals and 9 key books on medicine, nutrition and health.

0-595-29675-0